Understanding Mild Traumatic Brain Injury (MTBI)

An Insightful Guide
To Symptoms, Treatments and
Redefining Recovery

Based on *Mild Traumatic Brain Injury:
A Survivor's Handbook*
by Theta Theta No Beta

Edited by

Mary Ann Keatley, PhD, CCC
and Laura L Whittemore

A Brain Injury Hope Foundation Publication

Brain Injury Hope Foundation
P. O. Box 1319
Boulder, CO 80306

Telephone: 303-484-2126
www.BrainInjuryHopeFoundation.org

Proceeds from book sales go to the Brain Injury Hope Foundation, a nonprofit organization in Boulder, Colorado that provides emergency financial assistance to individuals with MTBI in Colorado. The Foundation's mission is also to promote awareness and understanding of mild traumatic brain injury through publications and presentations.

Disclaimer: This book is not designed to replace a physician's independent judgment about the appropriateness or risks of a procedure or therapy for a given patient. Our purpose is to provide you with information and understanding that will help you make confident health care decisions.

Cover design by Tony Greco
www.tonygrecodesign.com

Interior illustrations by Kersti Frigell
kfrigell@comcast.net

Photos by Barbara Colombo
www.11-11productions.com

Interior design by Ronnie Moore
westype@comcast.net

Library of Congress Control Number: 2010922023
ISBN: 978-0-9824094-1-1

Printed in the United States of America

*This book is dedicated to the strength and courage
of the survivors of brain injury who
are the unrecognized heroes
who persevere to
recover and
thrive.*

Acknowledgments

We wish to acknowledge that this book was inspired by a small handbook entitled, *Mild Traumatic Brain Injury: A Survivor's Handbook*, written by Theta Theta No Beta, a Colorado based MTBI support group and edited in 1995 by Robin Murphy Davis. Robin was one of the original authors of the Survivor's Handbook and a beloved member of our community. She was a member of the Brain Trust and an inspiration to all those she touched.

The name Theta Theta No Beta is a reference to brain waves. Those suffering from MTBI often have an increase in theta waves and a decrease in beta waves. Members of Theta Theta No Beta are Leana Bowman, Maurene Flory, Lori Maki, Bhadra Mitchell, Lesley Reed, Connie Scribner, Robin Murphy Davis, Judith Frans, Maria

Michael, Laura Phillips, Carol Roberts, and Katy H. Wolf. Their efforts to produce the book were encouraged and supported by Mary Lou Acimovic, MA, CCC-Sp, who contributed expertise and editorial assistance throughout the process; and Jan Lemmon, PhD, who shared her knowledge and scholarly advice about brain injury.

The Survivor's Handbook was updated in 2006 by The Brain Trust, a nonprofit organization, now known as the Brain Injury Hope Foundation (BIHF), based in Boulder, Colorado. Donald Davis generously licensed the Survivor's Handbook to the Brain Injury Hope Foundation to publish, modify, reorganize, transform, distribute and sell. Proceeds from book sales go to the Brain Injury Hope Foundation to promote awareness and understanding of brain injury and to provide emergency financial assistance to survivors of mild to moderate traumatic brain injury in Colorado.

Thank you to Ricardo Esparza, PhD, for his support and technical expertise especially on the post traumatic stress disorder definition. A special thanks goes to Ronnie Lynn Moore, interior book designer, and to Tony Greco, book cover designer, and to Kersti Frigell, interior illustrator, for donating a large portion of their time and expertise because they believed in our vision. Thank you to Karen

Carpenter, MA, CCC-A, who provided technical assistance on the hearing section; to Lisa Lanzano, MS, RD, who contributed a major portion of nutrition chapter and Joanne Phillips who contributed her knowledge of neutraceuticals that enhance brain function. Thank you to Rebecca Hutchins, OD, FCOVD, who assisted with the vision chapter; and to Lisa Kreber, PhD, for her expertise on physical exercise and brain injury. Thank you to Ty Miller, L.Ac., who provided the definition of acupuncturist and to Judy Haddow, MA, CCC, for her help in editing and valuable input. Thank you to Carol Schneider, PhD, and Diane Coffelt for their editing/ proofreading suggestions as well as to Suzanne Brackley for editing the legal and insurance chapter.

As you can see there were many MTBI survivors and health care professionals who felt compelled to provide a better understanding of the symptoms and the recovery process of brain injury. Those who went before will be proud to know that their message of hope inspired us to write and edit this book. It is our intention to create a greater awareness and compassion that will provide a positive environment for healing.

Table of Contents

Traumatic Brain Injury has been labeled the "Silent Epidemic."

CHAPTER 1

Understanding Mild Traumatic Brain Injury (MTBI)

It happens in the blink of an eye. In that instant your life is changed. It may have been caused by a fall, automobile or sports related accident or a blast injury from an explosion. Recovering from mild traumatic brain injury (MTBI) is a new experience not only for those who are injured but also for those caring people who want to help. The first step is to learn all you can about MTBI and to accept it as a starting point—a new beginning.

This book was created for you, your family, and your support system to increase awareness about brain injuries. It is our intention to empower you with the inside knowledge and wisdom gained from those who experienced MTBI and moved through the healing process, in order to survive, thrive and ultimately prevail in their lives.

Although mild traumatic brain injury affects millions of people and was recognized well over a hundred years ago, it is currently taking a position in the limelight. Numerous articles and TV specials are covering the effects of TBI on our Wounded Warriors returning from Iraq and Afghanistan. Many professional athletes are stepping forward to report the possible long-term affects from multiple concussions.

Use this book as a guide to navigate through the unknown territory of brain injury. What you are experiencing may be unknown to you and your loved ones, and it is also a new frontier in science and research. The innovations in science, computers and imaging are moving at lightening speed at the same time that there appears to be an acknowledge-ment and acceptance of this type of injury. Basically, we have a perfect cataclysm of science and humanity coming together to advance research and help solve the mysteries of brain injury and open new doors for recovery.

The ideas presented in this book are recommendations. It is essential that you consult a professional to develop a treatment program that is individually designed for your needs. Your brain is one of your most important assets and it is worth rehabilitating to improve the quality of your life.

Definition of MTBI

A mild traumatic brain injury (MTBI) is defined as a blow or jarring of the head that results in a disruption of brain functioning. MTBI has been labeled the "Silent Epidemic"[1] Brain injuries can range from "mild" to "severe." All brain injuries should be considered serious, and you should alert your physician about the symptoms you are having.

Mild traumatic brain injuries are usually called "closed head injuries" because there is a non-penetrating injury to the brain. This type of injury can be caused by whiplash, a blast injury, or hitting the head, resulting in bruising, stretching, and shearing of the axons and/or tearing of the tissues. For the complete medical definition of MTBI, refer to Appendix A.

Contrary to popular belief, you DO NOT need to hit your head to sustain a mild traumatic brain injury. A whiplash injury, where the head accelerates and decelerates without making contact, can cause a brain injury. There is also new research that indicates that concussions may be caused by blast waves from explosions. Studies being done at Johns Hopkins reveal that even if you were not hit in the head or knocked out, the indirect, powerful pressure waves caused by a bomb may affect the brain.[2]

MTBI Often Goes Unidentified or Misdiagnosed

Many times the brain injury is not documented during the acute stage, because physical pain overrides the awareness of MTBI. Following a concussion or MTBI, awareness levels may be reduced and you may not realize that you have suffered a brain injury. As the body begins to heal and you become more active, the head injury becomes more apparent.

The history of mild traumatic brain injury has been documented for more than a century. During the 1860s, it was discovered that individuals who were injured in railway collisions suffered from brain injuries. It was believed that their symptoms were caused by "nervous shock" to the spinal cord and the brain.[3] More recent research notes that the symptoms of mild brain injury are much more serious than previously believed or shown through testing.[4]

The latest report from the Center for Disease Control (CDC) states that approximately 1.7 million people sustain a brain injury in the United States each year, and 800,000 of those are believed to be mild traumatic brain injuries. TBIs are increasing among children because of their involvement in sports.

The CDC also reports that 1.1 million are treated and released from emergency departments, but the actual number of people with TBI, who are not seen in emergency rooms or do not receive care, is unknown. An estimated 5.3 million Americans are living with TBI related disabilities. The greatest number of traumatic brain injuries are caused by falls followed by motor vehicles accidents.

Brain injuries are cumulative in nature. In other words, if you suffer more than one concussive injury over time, the effects may accumulate and even a small impact to the head, may manifest as a more serious injury.

Neurological examinations and brain imaging studies, such as MRI and CT Scans, may be normal even if you have sustained a brain injury. However, your doctor may have ordered these tests in the beginning to rule out other medical conditions. Newer imaging tests, such as PET Scans or SPECT Scans, have proven to be more informative for this type of injury. The field of neuroimaging is changing rapidly so be sure to consult your doctor to determine which tests would be most beneficial.

Although the injury may be "invisible" to the outside observer, MTBI usually has a number of symptoms, such as nausea, dizziness, vomiting, sleep disturbance, blurred vision, sensitivity to light and sound, fatigue, etc. Emotionally you may feel a shaken sense of self and out of control. Very often there is an overlap of symptoms of Traumatic Brain Injury (TBI) and Post Traumatic Stress Disorder (PTSD).

My Thoughts and Observations

*A neuropsychological evaluation
from a neuropsychologist helps to delineate
symptoms of depression, PTSD and MTBI.*

CHAPTER 2

Post Traumatic Stress Disorder (PTSD)

Survivors of TBI are particularly susceptible to major depression, generalized anxiety disorder, and post-traumatic stress disorder.[1] PTSD frequently co-exists with mild traumatic brain injury and has many of the same symptoms. PTSD is defined as a disorder that develops after a distressing psychological event that is outside typical human experience. It is characterized by re-experiencing or reliving, over and over again, painful or stressful situations. Examples of traumatic emotional events that can cause PTSD include wars, accidents, physical and mental abuse and natural disasters (hurricanes, earthquakes). Even rescue workers and first responders, such as firefighters, EMTs and police may experience secondary traumatic stress disorder. Medical workers, such as ER doctors, nurses, psychologists, therapists and caregivers have been known to experience compassion fatigue.

The symptoms of PTSD may include nightmares, flashbacks, avoiding stimuli associated with the trauma, recurring memories, poor concentration, trouble sleeping, anger, exaggerated responses, and hypervigilance.

Since the symptoms of PTSD and MTBI can be very similar and may overlap, it is essential to identify all of your symptoms and receive appropriate treatments. A neuropsychological evaluation from a neuropsychologist helps to differentiate between the symptoms of PTSD and MTBI.

By looking at the symptoms and biology of trauma, we can begin to understand PTSD. In 1997 Dr. Peter Levine wrote a book entitled *Waking the Tiger: Healing Trauma*. In this book he talks about the body's reaction to threat and/or trauma. An individual may respond to a traumatic experience by fighting, fleeing or freezing.

Fight or flight responses are also known as acute stress responses. Dr. Levine reports that when an individual is threatened and their attempts to fight or flee seemingly fail, they may move into a freeze response, otherwise know as immobility. Also, if the energy that is created by this threatening situation is not discharged from the nervous system through fighting or fleeing, this can lead to more intense reactions of rage, helplessness or terror. When these feelings build up to a certain "level of activation that overwhelms the nervous system," the immobility or freeze response may take over.[2]

Signs of activation may include rapid, shallow breathing, rapid heart rate, muscle tension, and racing thoughts. Individuals who suffered brain injuries accompanied by post traumatic stress described these feelings of overwhelm and heightened startle responses to sound, light, smell and/or motion. For example, if you are already in a state of high activation, a simple knock on the door or someone walking up behind you can cause a significant startle response.

Hypervigilance is like being in the state of "intense alertness at all times..."[3] If an individual cannot identify the source of the threat, their internal response to what appears to be dangerous will continue and could possibly become amplified. This in turn may increase the intensity of the freeze response, and the person may become hypervigilant, perceiving or feeling danger in many situations where none exists.

An example of hypervigilance is when individuals with PTSD are triggered by a situation and perceive it as a threat. They identify the threat as coming from outside of themselves, when it is really an internal feeling of arousal. Even if the outside threat is identified and dealt with, the intensity of the internal arousal is so great that hypervigilant behaviors continue.

Recommended treatments for PTSD may include medication, psychological counseling, Eye Movement Desensitization and Reprocessing (EMDR), brain spotting, Somatic Experiencing, cognitive rehabilitation, and physical therapy.

My Thoughts and Observations

_____

_____

_____

_____

_____

_____

_____

_____

_____

_____

_____

_____

_____

_____

_____

_____

_____

_____

_____

_____

_____

_____

_____

There is nothing mild about
a mild traumatic brain injury.

CHAPTER 3

What Are the Signs and Symptoms of MTBI?

Brain injuries cause a constellation or group of symptoms that affect overall functioning. Heightened sensitivity to the environment is a common symptom of MTBI.

The following list of symptoms are often associated with MTBI:

Physical symptoms may include:
- Headaches
- Heightened awareness of physical aches and pains
- Nausea, vomiting
- Loss of balance
- Vision problems, blurred vision

- Difficulty reading
- Dizziness
- Loss of sex drive
- Loss of energy
- Easily fatigued
- Sensitivity to light, sound, touch
- Sleep disturbance
- Decrease in senses of smell and taste
- Difficulty with choking and swallowing

Emotional symptoms may include:

- Depression
- Mood swings
- Fearfulness
- Apathy, lack of interest, lack of concern
- Low motivation
- Gullibility
- Feeling easily overloaded
- Anxiety, frustration
- Difficulty managing emotions
- Hypervigilance, exaggerated startle response
- Sense of helplessness
- Loss of sense of self, low self-esteem
- Nightmares
- Anger, sudden outbursts
- Mania, excessive excitement

Cognitive or thinking symptoms may include:

- Memory loss, forgetting appointments
- Short attention span, easily distracted
- Slowed thinking and longer response time
- Disorientation, confusion
- Brain fatigue, feeling as if in a fog
- Forgetfulness, misplacing things, forgetting previously learned skills
- Difficulty driving, getting lost easily
- Inability to recall words
- Spelling difficulty
- Impaired comprehension, difficulty following conversations
- Difficulty thinking in noisy environments
- Inability to organize thoughts
- Inability to multitask, perform two or three things at once
- Inability to start or finish tasks
- Inability to inhibit certain behaviors—excessive shopping, gambling
- Difficulty with abstract thinking
- Inability to focus on reading, watching TV, computer tasks

For a more detailed self-assessment, please refer to the Functional Symptom Questionnaire in Appendix B. This questionnaire is a valid and reliable tool used to recognize typical symptoms caused by mild traumatic brain injury. It is extremely valuable in measuring your progress over time. Take this assessment tool now and again every 3 to 6 months to track your healing progress and to pinpoint areas that need attention. Remember, the healing process is unique to everyone and the physical, emotional, cognitive and thinking abilities improve at different rates.

Research completed on the questionnaire revealed that both MTBI and non-injured individuals reported their greatest problems occurred in the Attention/Concentration area. However, those with MTBI reported a higher incidence of concentration problems. Another interesting observation was that the second area of greatest difficulty for MTBI was in Emotional Functioning; whereas the second greatest difficulty for the non-injured group was Memory.

No matter where you are in your recovery, if you are experiencing any of the above symptoms, pay attention to the *frequency* and the *intensity* of a symptom. How often does it occur? Apply the frequency scale of Never, Sometimes, Frequently, or Almost Always to any symptom or behavior. For example, do you find yourself missing an appointment, getting confused, or losing your car keys more often than usual?

In addition to *frequency*, it is valuable to be aware of the *intensity* of a symptom or a behavior. For example, the *intensity* of the sound of a person's voice may be too loud or irritating. Very often, the background noise in a restaurant can be overwhelming and uncomfortable making it difficult to follow the conversations of the people that you may be dining with.

Common Symptoms of Cognitive-Communication Impairment

Many people have trouble thinking clearly following a traumatic brain injury. They sometimes say, "I feel like I am in a fog," or "It's like my brain shuts off and the thoughts won't come."

A clinical term for this type of difficulty is "cognitive-communication impairment." Cognition refers to the mental process of thought, as it relates to awareness, perception, thinking, reasoning and judgment. During the healing period, the brain fatigues rapidly and may shut down. This is called the "camera shutter effect." When the brain is rested, the shutter is open. Information comes in easily and can be filtered in terms of what warrants attention. When the brain becomes fatigued because of overload (e.g. too much sound or light, or too much cognitive effort) the shutter will close. You may see people's lips moving, but not understand what they are saying. You may also feel like your brain is tired and you need to rest.

Once your brain is ready, it is important to engage in cognitive rehabilitation. Cognitive therapy has been proven to be very effective in the rehabilitation of thought processes following a brain injury. Such therapy is usually done with a Speech-Language Pathologist or Occupational Therapist who specialize in the treatment of brain injuries.

If you had a mild traumatic brain injury, one theory of rehabilitation purports that your knowledge base and previous skills still exist. Cognitive rehabilitation provides tasks to re-stimulate those brain functions and allows the skills to re-emerge. This type of therapy restores thinking processes and helps them to become automatic again. For suggestions of simple memory and cognitive activities that you can do on your own, please read Chapter 11.

Computer programs that are specifically designed to improve cognitive and memory skills can be very helpful and yet represent only one of the many techniques used by an experienced provider who is up to date on the latest treatments. Be sure your provider is using a variety of exercises and is recommending other activities that improve brain functioning.

The following list of skills can be improved with cognitive and language rehabilitation:

- Memory (short term memory, long term memory, working memory, etc.)
- Concentration and Attention—auditory and visual attention
- Language and word retrieval—written and verbal
- Logic and reasoning skills—solving problems by defining options and making decisions
- Speed of information processing
- Flexibility of thinking—switching from one task to another or generating more than one solution to a problem
- Executive Functioning—self-initiation, planning, prioritizing, self-monitoring errors
- Organizational skills—developing systems for bill-paying, laundry, shopping
- Increasing awareness levels
- Reading, writing, basic math skills
- Pragmatic skills—conversational skills, when to talk, what to talk about, reading facial expressions of others

Since certain skills will take longer to recover, it may be necessary to develop compensatory strategies that can build on your strengths and work around deficits. Developing effective ways to compensate diminishes feelings of frustration and anxiety.

Remember, your thinking will improve and you will be able to tolerate more cognitive stamina as you recover. A common question asked is "Can just doing my job replace cognitive rehabilitation?" The answer is "not really," because work skills are usually over-learned behaviors and skills that were learned and repeated for a period of time. Rehabilitating the brain is best accomplished through learning to do new things. Novel mental and physical tasks, such as playing cognitive games, studying a new language, learning a musical instrument or dance steps, help to re-establish neural pathways. The repetition required by new learning helps to rewire and rehabilitate the brain. Read more about rewiring and neuroplasticity of the brain in Chapter 16.

Common Symptoms of Pain

Following a brain injury, it is normal to experience pain sensations in different parts of the body. Pain that originates in one part of the body, but causes pain in a different location is called "referred pain". For example, a neck injury may refer pain into the head or down into the back.

Pain can cause physical hurt as well as mental anguish that may range from mild to severe. Typical words used to describe the pain experience are sharp, dull, aching, burning and throbbing. The mental anguish caused by pain is a significant consequence that can negatively affect the quality of one's life. We recommend that you seek help, since there are many treatment options available.

The two primary types of pain are:

- **Acute Pain:** This pain can be very intense and last for a short time until the injury heals.
- **Chronic Pain:** Chronic pain lasts for at least three months and may occur for months or even years. Chronic pain can range from mild to severe.

It is sometimes difficult to measure pain with objective tests, but your doctor may ask questions and give you a questionnaire to rate the type, frequency and severity of the pain. Pain can occur in any part of the body. Some individuals report that their pain is worse if they sit for periods of time in certain positions; whereas others find that moving around increases their pain sensations.

Pain may disrupt your sleep, as well as your ability to think or perform cognitive/memory tasks. Prolonged pain may cause fear, depression, anxiety and anger. In Turk and Winter's book, *The Pain Survival Guide*,[1] they report many common chronic pain conditions, such as back pain, whiplash , fibromyalgia, migraine and tension headaches. Like brain injuries, your pain may be invisible to others, but very real to you. It is important not to over-analyze or question the reality of your pain, even if others infer that you are exaggerating.

It is important that you learn to manage your pain and not push beyond your physical limits. You will know when your body and brain are ready for more activity. Pay attention because you are the best judge of your limitations. Take it slow and easy. By being aware of your pain symptoms and developing psychological coping skills to deal with them, it facilitates the recovery process.

Common pain treatments include: rest, heat, ice, massage, physical therapy, osteopathic work, chiropractic treatments, biofeedback and relaxation, such as breathing exercises and visual imagery, acupuncture, hypnosis, ultrasound, electrical stimulation, changing your activity level, taking medications, injections and surgery. Consult your doctor to determine the best treatments for your specific pain symptoms. If you do not get relief, there are doctors who specialize in pain, and there are pain clinics that successfully treat chronic pain. Pain psychologists specialize in improving your mood and your pain, and provide stress management skills. Above all else, trust your feelings and function within your ability.

Common Symptoms of Headaches

Headaches are one of the most common symptoms of mild traumatic brain injuries. There are various causes and types of headaches associated with MTBI. Trauma to the head or whiplash injuries to the neck may cause post-traumatic headaches (PTH) and/or muscle tension headaches. Headache pain can be very debilitating and affect your daily functioning. Headaches can affect your ability to interact with your family, do your job, or engage in social and recreational activities.

Headaches are classified into several types and may range from mild to severe, and may be dull, sharp or throbbing. Some individuals describe their headaches as happening "24/7"; meaning that they have some degree of head pain all of the time, 24 hours per day, seven days a week. This is not uncommon following even the "mildest" of head injuries. We believe there is nothing mild about a mild traumatic brain injury.

Individuals may have more than one type of headache. They may experience a combination of tension, post-traumatic or other types of headaches. Undergoing a thorough examination and history will help your doctor identify the types, triggers and treatments for your headaches. It may be important to have both a general medical exam and a neurological evaluation of your headaches.

One common type of headache is called a *tension-type headache*. This may originate at the base of the skull or from excessive muscle tension in the neck, jaw, face or scalp. The pain associated with tension headaches has been described as dull or aching and may increase over the course of the day. Some people describe it as feeling like a "band around their head."

If you awaken in the morning with a tension headache, it could be related to clenching or grinding your teeth during the night, and it may be prudent to consult with a dentist who specializes in temporomandibular (TMJ) disorders. Dentists can fit you with a specialized mouth guard to wear at night to protect your teeth and relax the muscles, which in turn, may decrease or stop muscle tension headaches.

Another type of headache is called *posttraumatic migraine headache* or a vascular headache. This type of headache may be accompanied by or start with an aura or some type of visual symptom before the headache begins. An aura is usually a visual symptom, such as flashing or sparkling lights, lines in your visual fields, or your vision may be blotted out. Objects may seem farther away or closer. Some people have reported getting the aura without the migraine pain, which can be referred to as a silent migraine.

Other brain-related symptoms may occur, such as numbness on one side of the face or hand, weakness, and unsteadiness. The aura can be used as a signal that you need to lie down and rest, take medications, or use an ice pack on the back of your head or neck to diminish the severity.

Biofeedback is a nonpharmacological treatment for both tension headaches and migraine headaches. A more thorough explanation of Biofeedback can be found in Chapter 12 "What Is Biofeedback and Neurofeedback?" If posttraumatic headaches persist, ask your physician or neurologist about medications to help alleviate the pain and break the headache cycle. It is important to have education and support to deal with headaches associated with MTBI.

A multidisciplinary approach for the treatment of headaches may include an evaluation with a doctor, and treatment with a physical therapist, biofeedback therapist, and counselor, as well as an assessment of your need for medications.

Effects of Barometric Pressure and Altitude

You may also notice that weather patterns or elevation changes may intensify your headaches, pain and other physical symptoms. Some people will take a vacation at sea level, in order to take a "vacation" from their headaches. The correlation between high altitude and headaches has been well documented.[2]

When changes in barometric pressure occur, individuals with MTBI complain of headaches intensifying, especially when storms move in and the barometer drops. Some countries are on the cutting edge of weather-based health forecasts that alert people to barometric pressure changes. For example, Canada has on-line services that forecast barometric changes. For more information go to their website www.ec.gc.ca/Envirozine.[3]

Once you are aware of the frequency and intensity of your symptoms, you can alter the environment you are in and/or your behaviors to help manage your recovery.

Remember that some symptoms can be increased by medications. You may also have side effects resulting from medications. If you have questions, discuss them with your doctor as soon as possible.

Common Symptoms of Fatigue

Many individuals complain of fatigue following traumatic brain injury that may occur only in the beginning phases of recovery or it may last up to several years or more. Typical statements made by patients about fatigue include: "I'm so exhausted I don't want to get out of bed." "I feel like I'm in a fog, like I can't make myself think." "I'm so tired that I can't make my brain process information."

Researchers have studied various types of fatigue, including mental or cognitive fatigue, physical fatigue and psychological fatigue. Recent research studies show that fatigue is present in up to 73% of individuals who suffer TBI, and is the first symptom reported by many individuals.[4] Physical fatigue may occur from having to work harder to perform physical tasks, such as cleaning the house or working around the yard. Physical fatigue becomes worse over the day and is usually helped by rest or sleep.

Mental or cognitive fatigue may occur when you put forth cognitive effort, such as trying to concentrate, read, balance your checkbook, or solve problems. You may have been able to do these things automatically before your brain injury, but now they may take greater effort, and your accuracy and efficiency may have decreased. Psychological fatigue is related to stress and/or depression. This type of fatigue is worse in the morning and is not usually helped by sleep.

Following are some recently documented facts about fatigue and head injury:

- Fatigue is usually greater in the early months following your injury.
- Mental fatigue, followed by physical fatigue, are the most prominent types of fatigue following traumatic brain injury.[5]
- Mental fatigue after MTBI can be "profoundly disabling and affect working capacity as well as social activities."[6]
- Fatigue following a brain injury has "significant impact on well-being and quality of life."[7]
- Individuals have complained about fatigue following head injury for many years. But, recent research now confirms that fatigue is real and affects one's ability to mentally process information. Objective studies show that fatigue causes slower speed of information processing and difficulties with attention.[8]

- Functional MRIs are used to objectively assess cognitive fatigue in persons with TBI compared to healthy controls.[9]

Because fatigue significantly impacts a person's functioning following a brain injury, more researchers are studying it and using fatigue scales, such as the Fatigue Severity Scale and Causes of Fatigue Questionnaire to assess a person's level of fatigue. Researchers are using more objective measures to find molecular mechanisms, such as abnormal protein markers, abnormal pituitary functions (hypopituitarism) and hormonal deficiencies as a result of MTBI. Since 25 to 50% of those individuals studied had problems with pituitary function, early screening for this problem is highly recommended.[10] These tests may help explain the long-lasting effects of fatigue following MTBI. Other research is also documenting the potential role of glutamate transport in mental fatigue.[11] Perhaps in the near future, successful treatments will be available to boost energy levels and decrease the devastating effects of fatigue. Medications, adequate nutritional intake, and increased rest are common treatments. Consult your care providers for the latest information in this area.

You Don't Know What You Don't Know

When the brain is injured, it has to protect itself by shutting out stimuli from the outside world. In other words, the brain shuts down. This may happen many times in an hour or in a day. Sometimes individuals don't recognize the symptoms of traumatic brain injury, but when they start to recover from their physical injuries, they often say, "I was so injured that I wasn't aware of what I was doing or saying."

At such times, your awareness levels may be low. It is difficult to know what you are missing until the brain starts to heal and the "cloud lifts."

Before an injury, many skills came automatically but after the injury, you may have forgotten certain parts of a skill. Previously, you did not have to give full attention to certain activities, such as cooking, reading a book, working on the computer, or driving to familiar places. After a brain injury the "automatic pilot" may or may not be functioning efficiently and your speed of processing can be much slower. Although you think you know how to do a task, you might be surprised to find out that the body is willing but the brain is slower to respond. In other words, "You don't know what you don't know." Don't be embarrassed or fearful. Rely on people whom you trust as you move through the early stages of healing.

My Thoughts and Observations

"The most effective thing is not getting hit in the first place," says Harvard quarterback Vin Ferrara in a *Time* magazine interview.

CHAPTER 4

Sports-Related Concussions

Concussions or mild traumatic brain injuries (MTBI) are sometimes called "dingers," "bell ringers," "seeing stars" or being "punch drunk." Although motor vehicle accidents and falls are responsible for significantly more head and brain injuries than sports, the U.S. Centers for Disease Control (CDC) and Prevention estimates "1.6 to 3.8 million sports-related TBIs occur each year" as a result of all types of sports and recreational activities.[1]

There was previously a misconception in contact sports, such as football and boxing, that helmets fully protected a person from sustaining a brain injury. According to TIME Magazine (February 2010), "Helmets do a nice job of protecting the exterior of the head and preventing deadly skull fractures. But, concussions occur within the cranium, when the brain bangs against the skull. When helmets clash, the head decelerates instantly, yet the brain can lurch forward, like a driver who jams the brakes on."[2] This can cause bruising of the brain and stretching of tissues.

Repeated blows to the head can cause a cumulative effect, and have "lifelong repercussions." It is a known fact that 19% of NFL players between the ages of 30 and 49 are "debilitated." The chance of having a memory-related diagnosis such as Alzheimer's or dementia is 1 in 53 in NFL players compared to 1 in 1000 in the general population of men 30 to 49 years of age.

The term coined to describe these repeated blows is "chronic traumatic encephalopathy (CTE)."[3] According to Dr. Ann McKee of Boston University School of Medicine, there is a build up of the protein called "tau", which becomes toxic in neurodegenerative diseases such as Alzheimer's, and is found only in individuals with CTE or other neuro-degenerative diseases.

In normally functioning individuals it is found in only limited amounts. Dr. McKee notes that this "unique pattern of changes" in tau proteins is only seen "in this severity" in individuals who have a history of repetitive head trauma, including boxers and football players. Dr.

McKee asks that "radical steps" be taken to change the way football is played, and to make those changes today.

Brain injuries caused by sports related activities have oftentimes been assessed using different parameters than those caused by motor vehicle accidents or slip and falls. One primary question regarding recreational sports injuries focuses on when the individual can safely return to the game.

In December 2009, the NFL issued new, more stringent, guidelines regarding the nature and severity of concussive symptoms that require immediate removal from the game. These include such things as amnesia, poor balance and abnormal neurological examinations. These do not necessarily include dizziness or headaches. One positive aspect is that physicians, coaches and players are using a more critical eye regarding MTBI associated with sports activities, not only in the major sports leagues, but at the college and high school levels.

The Leading Cause of Sports-Related Injuries

The incidence of individuals who went to hospital emergency departments due to sports-related and recreation-related, non-fatal brain injuries were studied by the CDC. They analyzed data from the National Electronic Injury Surveillance System from 2001-2005.

Following are the leading causes of sports-related injuries in the order of reported incidence:

- Bicycling
- Football
- Playground
- Basketball
- All-terrain vehicles
- Baseball
- Soccer
- Horseback riding
- Swimming/diving
- Skateboards
- Hockey

It should be noted that the incidence seen in emergency departments may differ from the number and severity of injuries seen by athletic trainers, who deal primarily with contact sports.[4]

Dr. James Kelly and Dr. Jay Rosenberg wrote guidelines for the management of sports-related concussions for the Colorado Medical Society as early as 1990, and they addressed the need for consultation with an independent, "well-informed physician" to help prevent catastrophic outcome from repeated concussions.[5]

There is an increasing awareness of the seriousness of all injuries to the brain, and The American Academy of Neurology reports that "there is no such thing as a minor concussion." The American Academy of Neurology published specific guidelines based on those of Kelly and Rosenberg, to assess concussions in all types of athletic activities. It is a known fact that, "Any sport has an inherent risk of injury. A balance must be reached between maintaining a competitive edge in a sport and ensuring participant safety." Closely observing the injured athlete during the initial phases following the injury can be critical "to the prevention of a catastrophic brain injury."[6] In the same article, guidelines are documented regarding when an individual can return to competition following an injury.

The Grades of Concussions

Following are the three Grades of Concussions which classify the levels of severity of concussions.

- **Grade I**
  1. Transient confusion
  2. No loss of consciousness
  3. Concussion symptoms or mental status abnormalities on examination **resolve in** *less* **than 15 minutes**

- **Grade II**
  1. Transient confusion
  2. No loss of consciousness
  3. Concussion symptoms or mental status abnormalities on examination **last more than 15 minutes**

- **Grade III**
  1. Any loss of consciousness, either brief (seconds) or prolonged (minutes)

Grade I concussions are the most common, but are the most difficult to recognize because the individual does not lose consciousness and may only have momentary confusion or decreased concentration. In Grade II concussions, the athlete still does not lose consciousness, but their mental status examinations, poor concentration and/or lack of awareness lasts more than 15 minutes. If symptoms last an hour, this warrants medical observation. Grade III concussions are less difficult to recognize because the athlete is unconscious, and this can last for any length of time. With this level of concussion they are taken from the field to the emergency room.

The Practice Parameters for the management of concussions gives the following information: a detailed outline of the definitions of the various Grades of Concussions, features and symptoms of concussions, criteria for sideline evaluations, and recommendations for returning to the game.[7]

The Centers for Disease Control and Prevention (CDC) have developed a tool kit for coaches to reduce the number of sports concussions. This kit is called "Heads Up: Concussion in High School Sports." The kit contains practical, easy-to-use information including a video, DVD, posters, fact sheets for parents and athletes in both English and Spanish. They also advise, "It's better to miss one game than the whole season." Refer to their website for more information about youth in sports, and to order the kit go to www.cdc.gov.

Athletes should consider the "risk for second impact syndrome." This describes the concept that in a variety of sports, "once a person suffers a concussion, he is as much as four times more likely to sustain a second one."[8] It is also known that second impacts may require more time to recover. According to a New York Times article, *Girls Are Often Neglected Victims of Concussions*, high school girls playing soccer sustain 68% more concussions than boys, and girls playing basketball suffer almost three times the rate of concussions than high school boys.[9]

Can Concussions Affect Intelligence?

Discover Magazine explored whether contact sports can lower intelligence. Many studies have been done to measure the cognitive effects of soccer due to the "headers" that are performed when players hit the ball with their heads. The force of a soccer ball has been equated with the blows that boxers take to the head. Studies from many countries have substantiated that "the more someone heads a soccer ball, the lower that player will score on tests measuring attention, concentration, and general intellectual functioning"[10]

Among new innovations in sports safety are high-tech helmets worn by players, with embedded sensors used to measure g-forces that a player's head experiences upon impact. The new system is called HITS (Head Impact Telemetric System). The sensor in the helmet records the hit, which is sent to a computer on the sideline and documents the player's number and the magnitude of impact. It is hoped that this information can lead to better guidelines for evaluating sports related head injuries and the biomechanics involved.[11]

A number of years ago, Stuart Zatlin, a father, whose 12-year old son complained of dizziness after heading a fast-moving ball, invented a "laminated foam headband" called a "shinguard for your head" which reportedly softens the impact of headers by 30 to 50%.[12] There has been great controversy about wearing head gear or even padding the goal posts in soccer. Hopefully, the future will bring innovations to the sports fields, and new rules will be developed to provide a safe environment for the players of all ages. However, "The most effective thing is not getting hit in the first place," says Harvard quarterback Vin Ferrara in a TIME Magazine interview.[13]

Just imagine what it would be like with no filter on your brain. All the sounds, smells, images, and feelings would come crashing in at the same time.

CHAPTER 5

The Important Role of Brain Filters

Much of the brain's energy is used to filter out irrelevant or unnecessary information. Just imagine what it would be like with no filter on your brain. All the sounds, smells, images, and feelings would come crashing in at the same time. The overstimulation would probably paralyze you and prevent you from taking any action.

After sustaining MTBI, most of the brain's energy is diverted to basic functioning and little is left over for filtering or censoring. Trivial or insignificant thoughts often have the same weight in your mind as important ones. This can make decisions difficult. You may find that your brain gets stuck on an idea or phrase that keeps replaying, and this uses a great deal of brain energy.

New sensitivities can be very challenging and baffling for the injured person and their loved ones. Going into a restaurant or store where there are fluorescent lights, background music, or a great deal of visual stimuli may cause the brain to shut down. Most people say that they want to get into a quiet place and rest their brain. This is why it is so important to plan your social activities when fewer people are around and when there is less commotion. Even in a quiet room, small sounds such as a ticking clock seem to increase in volume over time.

Hearing Problems and Hypersensitivity to Sound

As mentioned above, a common symptom of traumatic brain injury is hypersensitivity to sound. This is called hyperacusis. The auditory system becomes very sensitive to environmental noise, and you may discover that you have great difficulty going to restaurants, the grocery store, or social gatherings.

Many individuals report staying at home to avoid the assault and the feelings of being overwhelmed in these noisy situations, or they may go out only at times when places are less crowded and less noisy. Any noise can irritate and overwhelm a person with MTBI, including a vibrating refrigerator, heating system or a humming fan.

An excellent accommodation for hyperacusis is the use of ear filters. One option is a custom-fitted earplug called, ER 15/25 noise-dampening ear filters which are very effective. They were originally made for musicians, but they are now being adapted for individuals with traumatic brain injuries. Consult an audiologist at a speech and hearing clinic to obtain filters. Another option for high-tech earplugs, which are being used by soldiers in the military, is the HearPlugz-DF.

Current studies show that filters can reduce overstimulation to the auditory system and allow you to participate in social situations without becoming overwhelmed. An advantage of using ear filters is that you can put them in for brief periods of time and take them out when you don't need them. They can be made with clear materials and are therefore less visible. The ear molds for these filters are made by an audiologist, or a specialist trained in testing hearing and treating hearing problems.

Some individuals suffer from tinnitus which is the perception of sound in the head when outside sound is not present. This is typically referred to as ringing in the ears. It may occur in one or both ears and may be caused by head and/or neck injuries. For additional information, contact the American Tinnitus Association, www.ata.org, or a local support group.

Vision Problems and Sensitivity to Light

You may notice that your eyes don't seem to be working in the same way that they did before your brain injury. Some eye doctors specialize in vision problems resulting from a traumatic brain injury. They can help diagnose visual problems related to the injury and provide vision therapy exercises or special glasses to help with recovery.

Because the visual changes are sometimes subtle, you may pass them off as being related to fatigue or brain fog. Aiming and focusing the eyes are linked, and that is why objects may appear to move, be seen as double, or blur in and out. Some individuals also complain that it is difficult to focus quickly from near to far or far to near.

Vision problems and cognitive deficits may compound one another. The most common complaints related to visual problems associated with brain injuries include light sensitivity, headaches, double vision, fatigue, dizziness, difficulty reading, or loss of peripheral visual fields. You may feel a heightened sensitivity to light and may even need to wear your sunglasses inside. You may have to request that fluorescent lights be turned off. Computer and reading tasks may take longer than usual and tend to be more confusing and tiring.

A behavioral optometrist or a doctor who belongs to the Neuro-Optometric Rehabilitation Association can perform a comprehensive vision evaluation and help you determine the best course of action. Some individuals with visual deficits can benefit from specific lenses or prisms in their glasses and/or from vision therapy.

If you have vision problems associated with MTBI, this may deplete your energy and decrease your ability to perform daily living tasks. It is unrealistic to return to work until vision problems are addressed. If your job requires a great deal of reading or moving your eyes between the desk and a computer screen, you may find that your errors increase because of difficulty tracking. It is very important to address visual problems, as they can increase the recovery time.

Dizziness and Vertigo

Feelings of dizziness and nausea are common after a head injury. You may notice that these symptoms come and go depending on the activity you are doing. Vertigo frequently occurs following MTBI and is the sensation of feeling as though you are spinning, and sometimes you feel nauseated or like you may lose your balance. Researchers have discovered various causes for this symptom, such as problems with your inner ear, impairments in eye movements, clenching and grinding your teeth or tightness in the neck muscles.

Dizziness may also originate from cervical neck injuries. The primary symptoms with this type of dizziness include feeling off balance, lightheadedness, and the sensation of floating. If you have what is called benign paroxysmal positional vertigo (BPPV), you may notice that you have a sudden attack of spinning when you turn over in bed, change your head position quickly, or reach for an item above your head. This usually lasts for less than a minute, but you may be left with feelings of nausea and dizziness for a longer time.

The Mayo Clinic developed a technique called canalith repositioning, where the head is maneuvered in various positions to help eliminate the dizziness. This is accomplished by moving the calcium crystals in the inner ear.[1] Medications that can help dizziness are also available. Be sure to consult with your doctor to see if you need a referral to an ear doctor who specializes in traumatic dizziness and/or an eye doctor who specializes in Post-Trauma Vision Syndrome.

Changes in Energy Reserve After Injury

Healing takes a tremendous amount of energy. The diagram in Figure 1 illustrates functioning before and after the injury. It shows how the uninjured brain can perform many activities that are physical, cognitive and emotional throughout the day, and still have a reserve of energy. After a brain injury, it takes more energy to deal with cognitive and emotional issues leaving little or no reserve.

The brain uses more energy than any other organ in the body. Before you were injured, you had a pool of reserve energy available when you overextended yourself. Following your injury, nearly all of your energy is required to perform the most basic functions just to get through the day. If you are continuing to work, you may find that when you get home, you must rest and not engage in other activities as before.

Figure 1. The Energy Pie

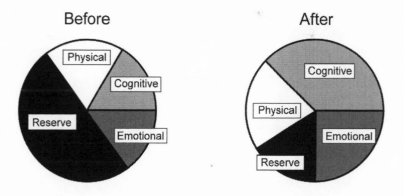

© Mary Lou Acimovic, MA, CCC-Sp

Your energy reserves at this point are almost nonexistent. When you push too much you may reach overload, and the extreme fatigue may cause your brain and body to shut down. This exhaustion can also amplify all of your symptoms and cause an emotional reaction.

Almost immediately after an injury it becomes clear that you don't have the same amount of energy that you previously did. It is important to emphasize the need for rest and conserving energy. For a while you may be unable to do as much as you used to and may need to take time out for rest—Brain Rest. Lie down during the day for naps. Even if you don't sleep, resting your head and lying down can make a significant difference in your recovery.

My Thoughts and Observations

*Most likely, your brain may be processing
more slowly, and the mechanisms that you could
previously depend on as your "automatic pilot"
may be temporarily damaged or not there
to protect you as they did before.*

CHAPTER 6

Baby, You Can Drive My Car

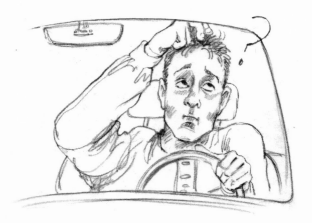

Regardless of whether your injury was caused by a motor vehicle accident or sports-related activity, it may take time before you feel comfortable behind the wheel. This is typical. The speed of traffic, the confusing activity in your peripheral vision, and the hypervigilant effort necessary for driving can overwhelm you. Being so overwhelmed can cause stress, increase headaches, and affect your reaction time. Some individuals report that it is even more difficult for them to ride as a passenger than to drive.

It is important to note again, "You don't know what you don't know"—meaning that you may think you are still capable of driving but discover that you should postpone driving for a while. For example, when you come to a four-way stop sign, you may forget what to do. Or, you might notice that when your eyes leave the road and you glance from left to right, you may get distracted longer than usual. Please pay attention to your level of awareness. Take a family member or a friend for a ride for a second opinion. Avoid driving when you are tired!

Most likely, your brain may be processing more slowly, and the mechanisms that you could previously depend on as your "automatic pilot" may be temporarily damaged or not there to protect you as they did before. It may be unsafe to do two things at the same time, such as driving while looking at the scenery, talking on a cell phone or to a passenger. This is a perfect example of multitasking skills that were previously taken for granted.

Your brain may struggle to register all the necessary infor-mation that driving requires. This previously occurred at lightning speed without much conscious thought. Now, processing may occur in a slower fashion. It is possible that you might find yourself lost while driving in an area you've known for years. If this happens to you, this might be another good reason to hand your car keys to someone else for a while.

Many individuals carry their cell phones with them while driving in case they have to PULL OVER to call someone to help orient them to their location or give them directions. You may also benefit from a GPS locator system that gives verbal directions.

Safety is of primary importance—yours, your passengers, and other drivers on the road. It is difficult to give up independence to drive where we want and when we want. The good news, though, is that this is probably temporary and you will be back behind the wheel in no time. Below are suggestions to consider during this transition time:

- Arrange to ride with a friend.
- Ask a friend to drive you in your car.
- Check out the bus routes.
- Use taxicabs or use demand-responsive transportation.
- Use roads that are less crowded, and don't drive during rush hour. It may take longer, but you will feel safer.

- Map out your route in advance, even if you have driven this route many times. It will be one less step for your brain to worry about.
- Explore the possibility of carpooling to your care providers with other patients. If you can coordinate appointments with another person, you can alternate driving and have company on the ride.
- Explore facilities in your area that specialize in teaching driving strategies to individuals who are returning to the road after an accident or physical injury. They can check out your reaction time.

My Thoughts and Observations

Appearances can be deceiving. You are dealing with a different person even though that person may look the same. Be compassionate, supportive, and patient.

CHAPTER 7

Helpful Tips for Family Members and Caregivers

Understanding mild traumatic brain injury is an important key to being successful in helping your loved one during the recovery process. This is also a time to take care of yourself. In communicating with many patients and families over the years it has become clear that everyone wants to be helpful but it is difficult to know the best actions to take. The most important key is to become educated about the injury. You can do this by reading or talking with the care providers. It is important to let your family member know that you understand their injury and that you believe them. Because it is an invisible injury, it is difficult to understand that your family member cannot perform in the way they could before. Avoid telling the injured person that they "look fine." Appearances can be deceiving. You are dealing with a different person even though that person may look the same. Be compassionate, supportive, and patient.

Be prepared for emotional mood swings, low energy and absentmindedness. Being compassionate and patient is very important.

One key symptom of MTBI is an inability to initiate actions. For example, the injured person may know what they want to do, know the steps to complete the task, but find that they are unable to physically begin. This is known as a "lack of initiation." It is very confusing and people sometimes mistake it for laziness or a lack of motivation. By understanding the nature of this symptom, there are rehabilitation techniques to break through the inability to get started.

Another symptom that oftentimes occurs is the inability to inhibit certain behaviors. This can occur during conversations when something unusual is said that would be uncharacteristic of the person. Another example of the inability to inhibit certain behaviors is when your family member spends money impulsively but does not realize it and has a lack of insight regarding the overall financial impact. Be sure to monitor spending habits and participate in balancing the checkbook to avoid overdrawn accounts.

You will probably have to do more than ever before. The injured person may find that even simple tasks will seem too much for them some days. Helping with errands and household chores, dealing with insurance companies and offering to drive them to appointments can make a world of difference. Try not to set any limits on recovery. Throw out the old schedule, forget old expectations, and embrace the person the way they are right now. Give them the space they need to heal and encourage your loved one to talk with others who understand.

You may also find it helpful to speak with others who have gone through this before. By talking with a counselor or care providers for your loved one, you may gain some insights about the recovery process. Do take care of yourself by taking personal time to recharge and renew your energy. Pace yourself throughout the day and pay attention to your own needs. Ask family and friends to share daily activities such as driving to appointments and running errands. Others want to be helpful, but oftentimes don't know how they can help. By allowing others to participate, you are giving them a gift as well.

Following are some helpful hints:

- **Structure the Day:** A regular routine minimizes the need for the person with the injury to rely on motivation and self-initiation of behaviors. If the day is left unstructured, there is a greater possibility that secondary problems will develop, such as confusion, depression, and anxiety.

- **Breakdown Activities into Small Steps:** A series of small, easily accomplished steps is less overwhelming to the injured individual than one big task. For example, decrease overload by making a grocery list the day before going to the store and then go to the store at a quiet time.

- **Recognize Fatigue and Be Flexible:** Positive outcomes are more likely when you move through the day within the physical, cognitive and emotional limitations of the individual. Pace activities throughout the day (e.g. one in the morning and one in the afternoon), alternating rest and activity. Since sleep cycles can often be disturbed, it is necessary to take naps to allow the brain and body to rest and maximize recovery.

- **Be Patient:** When an individual is healing from a brain injury, it is essential to allow them to move at their own pace. The brain processes information more slowly and it is best to allow the person adequate time to process auditory and visual information.

- **Simplify Your Explanations:** Use short phrases and repeat things in different ways to improve overall communication. It is also helpful to have a dry erase board or day planner in the home to write down activities, appointments, etc. This serves as a positive reminder and gives good visual cues so the person doesn't have to rely on their memory or others to remind them.

- **Use External Cues:** It is helpful to use a beeping reminder watch, cell phone alarm or talking watch that verbalizes the time as an external prompt for appointments. Various watches have multiple alarms that can be set throughout the day. These cueing devices can be gradually withdrawn as the individual is able to internally generate their own system of prompts, signals and reminders.

- **Communicate Simply and Sparingly:** Overstimulation (known as "hypersensitivity") from sound and light is a common symptom of brain injury. It is best to keep sound from the television and radio low, and keep conversation to a minimum. Humming noises from the refrigerator, computer, etc., frequently cause auditory overload. Turn lights down or off to help decrease light sensitivity. Fluorescent lights, such as in schools, offices and grocery stores, can trigger headaches.

- **Encourage Involvement:** Attending support groups of individuals with similar challenges can be very helpful. These groups provide education, social interaction, positive suggestions regarding recovery, and moral support. They can be helpful to the individual and the family. It is important to stay involved in social activities and stay connected with friends who understand.

- **Stay Positive But Realistic:** Everyone heals at their own rate from a brain injury. Because it can take a great deal of time to recover, it is important to emphasize and enjoy the activities the person can do rather than focusing on what they cannot do.

- **Help with Activities of Daily Living:** Assisting with bill paying, balancing the checkbook, and setting up appointments with doctors can be very helpful to the individual initially. This will help them conserve energy and get the rest that is critical for recovery. Once they are ready, encourage independence by helping to set up systems that the individual can follow through with on their own.

Focus on the little successes along the way, because with a hopeful heart you will see positive outcomes. In Appendix E, we have included "Helpful Questions for MTBI Survivors, Family Members, and Caregivers" that can be completed by the MTBI Survivor and can serve as an educational tool regarding ways to be helpful.

*Please know that you will get better,
you will learn to compensate and discover
your own resiliency and resourcefulness.*

CHAPTER 8

New Attitudes and Latitudes

Prior to your head injury, you may have been very self-sufficient. People came to you for help and now you are the one who could use some assistance. A typical response is to not want to impose, appear weak or feel obligated to others. Changing your attitude by asking for help may be new for you. Allowing people to help you is really a gift to them.

There may be times when you doubt the extent of your injury and try to continue your life as you did before. A natural reaction is to deny it, because you hope the symptoms will disappear. Denial is a form of self-protection and it is sometimes expressed as the numbing of feelings. It is a normal response to an abnormal situation. However, in the case of MTBI, if you don't move beyond this level of denial, you may miss the fast track to healing in those early months of recovery.

Biological changes in the brain associated with traumatic brain injury can coexist with psychiatric symptoms. In other words, these symptoms should be viewed from both a psychiatric and medical perspective. Among these are limbic rage which can occur because of the location of the injury, consequently setting off a cascade of hormones that cause an exaggerated expression of anger, an increased response to pain, and decrease in stress resiliency.

Balance and Structure

Create a new structure for your life. Plan your days and activities carefully. Set up a routine that works for you. Try not to overload yourself by scheduling too many things on any one day. Remember, activities that were easily accomplished before the accident, now require a great deal of planning and effort. Try to give yourself at least two or three "lighter load days" during the week.

You probably were able to do many things at the same time before your injury. Not being able to multitask is a common symptom of MTBI. For example, you may not be able to talk on the phone and cook dinner at the same time, talk and eat, drive a car, or even follow conversations.

Getting distracted, moving from one project to another and not completing things are examples of common symptoms following MTBI. People report feeling frazzled, confused and overwhelmed with the simple activities of daily life. That is why it is important to pace yourself and develop good time management skills by prioritizing tasks and limiting your activities. This will help to lower your frustration and anxiety levels immensely. Take a deep breath, relax and trust it will get better with time and recommended cognitive exercises.

If you are currently working or are considering returning to work, it may be important to let your supervisors and co-workers know what you are going through. Some individuals feel that it is important to protect the confidentiality around their injury and choose not to tell anyone. However, if there is a change in your performance, this information may help to gain their understanding and cooperation. The choice is yours. Another option is to take a leave of absence or assume less-complicated job responsibilities. Remember to plan a work schedule that allows time off for doctors appointments.

Sleep, Rest, and Sleep Some More

Oh, yes, sleep. Never before has sleep been so important. In the early stages of recovery, sleep may be what your

body and brain need most of all. Give in to it because
that is part of the natural healing response. Sleep as much
as you can, whenever and wherever you need to. Listen
to your body, and when it says it is tired, allow it to rest.

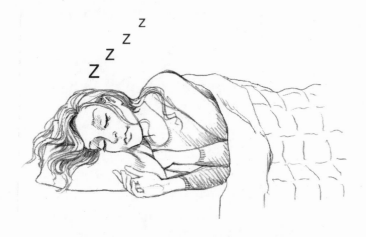

Plan on at least eight hours a night to allow your body
and mind to function at even the most basic level. Remember, you have little reserve energy—only a limited
amount each day—and that is greatly affected by how
much rest you have had.

However, you may have difficulties going to sleep or
experience sleep disruption as a result of the injury.
Consider taking naps throughout the day whenever you
feel tired. Explore ways to overcome this with your
healthcare providers.

Memory Tips

Maybe you used to keep lots of things in your head, but now you may find it extremely helpful to write down important information. Carry an appointment book, electronic or cell phone organizer with you. At home, keep a large, plain calendar in clear view in the kitchen or where you will see it frequently during the day. Refer to it several times during the day to remind you of the correct time of events and appointments. It's easy to get distracted and then confuse appointment times and dates, for example, showing up at the right time on the wrong day.

Don't force your brain to remember things that you can jot down on a "to do" list. It also might be helpful to write down directions to places you don't often go, such as medical providers, and keep them in your car.

Sometimes people feel disoriented to the time of day, and they use a beeping reminder watch or set their cell phone to alert them a half hour before an appointment.

A timer can be very helpful in reminding you when to take medications. Also setting the timer can prevent food from burning on the stove, and remind you that clothes are in the washing machine.

Special Assistive Devices

During the recovery process, it is important to use all means to make your life more comfortable. Assistive devices can help compensate for cognitive deficits, such as impaired memory or disorientation to time. These useful accessories range from simple appointment books and basic digital watches with multiple alarm functions to more advanced devices, such as watches that display reminder messages, for example "take medicine." There are also talking watches that tell the time of day. For more information about this watch and other assistive devices, go to www.Independentliving.com.

There are more complex devices with software packages that interface with a handheld PC. These provide reminders of events, maintain "to do" lists, and offer steps for sequencing daily tasks. For technical resources with cognitive support refer to www.ablelinktech.com

The following list of adaptive devices can make your life easier:

- Special earplugs to filter out unwanted noise, such as ER15/25 noise-dampening ear filters, noise-canceling headphones, or HearPlugz-DF (for the military, police & rescue workers)

- A dental mouth guard, or splint, to prevent damage to the teeth from clenching and grinding which can be used during the day or at night
- Lenses and filters for glasses to protect sensitive eyes including sunglasses and colored lenses

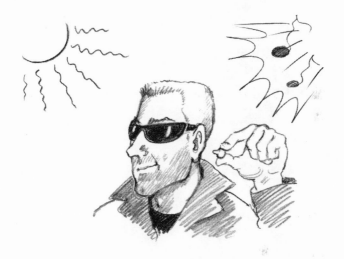

- Prism glasses to help when you are reading the computer screen
- Cushions to support the back and cervical spine
- Special pillows for sleeping
- Slant boards for use in reading
- Ergonomically correct chairs
- Talking Watch, timer or cell phone alarms as reminders for medications and appointments

- Hand-held devices that sync with computers
- Large, plain wall calendar
- Daily or weekly planner to keep track of appointments and necessary daily tasks
- Dry erase boards placed around the house to share messages between family members and/or communication notebooks to write down messages and confirm plans with family members
- Icepacks for the neck or back
- Orthotics (special shoe inserts)

My Thoughts and Observations

Having a coordinated treatment team and plan will expedite your recovery. Make sure your providers have expertise with brain injury.

CHAPTER 9

Medical Professionals Who Treat MTBI

For those with MTBI, recovery is a full-time job. The first part of that job is to find capable health care providers who understand MTBI. It is very important to choose a provider that you feel comfortable with and have confidence in their recommendations and treatment.

When choosing providers, be direct in asking questions such as, "Are you familiar with mild traumatic brain injury?" or "Have you had experience treating MTBI?" or "What is your approach in treating MTBI?" Based on their answers, you will have a better idea if this provider is right for you. Trust your instincts!

There are many kinds of therapists and doctors who can be helpful, however knowing where to go or who is best qualified to treat MTBI can be confusing. You may find that an interdisciplinary team of trained professionals is the best approach. The following list of health care providers will expand your awareness of the many options:

Doctors include:

- Primary care physician (PCP), such as a family doctor or an internist may be your first contact to obtain a diagnosis and prescribe ongoing care.
- Neurologists specialize in diagnosis and treatment of nervous system disorders, including diseases of the brain, spinal cord, nerves, and muscles.
- Osteopaths are physicians (DO) who take into account the physical, mental, emotional and spiritual health of a patient in their diagnosis. They use Osteopathic Manipulative Treatment to reduce pain.
- Chiropractors emphasize diagnosis, treatment and prevention of musculoskeletal disorders. Treatment may include adjustments, exercises, health and lifestyle counseling.
- Psychiatrists are physicians who specialize in diagnoses and medication management.
- Physiatrists are physicians who are experts in rehabilitation medicine and typically oversee the rehabilitation process.

- Naturopathic doctors (ND) practice as primary care providers of naturopathic medicine and emphasize the holistic approach. They use natural remedies such as herbs and foods.
- Ophthalmologists (MD) and Optometrists (OD) specialize in the diagnosis and treatment of Post-Trauma Vision Syndrome.

Therapists include:

- Psychologists, social workers, counselors, and coaches provide individual/marital/family counseling focused on developing coping skills, releasing trauma, and improving emotional, and social functioning.
- Physical therapists are health care professionals who provide hands-on mobilization and rehabilitative treatment to restore and maintain movement and function caused by injury.
- Speech-Language Pathologists can provide cognitive rehabilitation to help retrain your brain and improve memory through specific exercises as well as teach you ways to compensate for deficits while you recover.
- Occupational therapists evaluate and treat fine motor coordination and help strengthen independent living skills.

- Neuropsychologists perform extensive testing to evaluate brain-behavior relationships, plan rehabilitation strategies and document cognitive strengths and weaknesses.
- Massage therapists use manipulation of the soft tissue structures of the body to reduce stress and relax the body and mind.
- Craniosacral therapists use very light touch to relieve neck and back pain and balance the cranial sacral system of the body.
- Neurofeedback therapists use EEG biofeedback equipment to provide feedback about brain functioning and help to alter these frequencies and promote healing.
- Biofeedback specialists use sensitive instruments to measure physical responses, such as muscular tension, temperature, breathing, and fight-or-flight responses. They also provide feedback and strategies to retrain responses to stress.
- Acupuncturists insert needles the thickness of a fine hair into specific acupuncture points that are known to assist with rejuvenating the brain, calming headaches and relieving pain.
- Vision therapists help to correct and improve visual processing and perceptual disorders by

providing vision training with special eye exercises.

- Pilates instructors teach a series of non-impact exercises designed by Joseph Pilates to develop strength, flexibility, balance, and inner awareness.
- Vocational rehabilitation experts assist with exploring new vocations and retraining new job skills.
- Hypnotherapists help to modify behavior, habits, attitudes, anxiety, and help to manage pain.

Where to Start with Treatment Plans

Many health care professionals are not trained or familiar with the symptoms of MTBI. One starting point is to have a primary care physician (PCP) or a physiatrist with experience in MTBI to coordinate the types and timing of your treatments. Your doctor may refer you to a neurologist and a neuropsychologist for further evaluation.

Regardless of where you start, you will need to seek out care that is defined by the symptoms you have. Many individuals address the pain first by seeing an osteopathic physician or a physical therapist. Osteopathic physicians can provide craniosacral treatments to relieve headaches and pain. Acupuncturists also help decrease the intensity of aches and pains while physical therapists decrease pain, improve muscular strength and endurance. Hyperbaric oxygen is another treatment that individuals have found to be very helpful in the recovery process.

If you have difficulties thinking and remembering, contact a speech/language pathologist or occupational therapist who specializes in the treatment of cognitive problems associated with neurological disorders. You may need to see a neuropsychologist, who can evaluate, identify, and differentiate the cognitive symptoms from the emotional symptoms.

If trauma is a primary symptom, explore trauma release therapies, such as Eye Movement Desensitization and Reprocessing (EMDR), brain spotting, and Somatic Experiencing. These are performed by trained psychologists and counselors.

Optometrists who specialize in Post-Trauma Vision Syndrome offer vision therapy with eye exercises unique to your condition, or they may recommend special glasses to relieve pain or dizziness.

This is not an inclusive list. However, once you begin to see health care professionals who work with MTBI, they will direct you to others who will complement your treatment program. Again, it is important to stress that healing from a brain injury requires a multidisciplinary treatment program to meet all of your needs.

A Word about Medications

Medication is sometimes prescribed to decrease certain symptoms, such as pain, post-concussive headaches, dizziness, and depression. A Medication Record form is provided in Appendix C to help keep track of the names, dosages, and schedules of all medications. If you are taking supplements or herbal remedies, include them on your list. Take this record to share with your providers. Have your doctors and therapists talk with one another so that everyone is working together.

It is very important to eat healthy foods to help the brain function efficiently. Feed your brain with protein snacks throughout the day.

CHAPTER 10

Feed Your Body, Feed Your Brain: Nutritional Tips to Speed Recovery

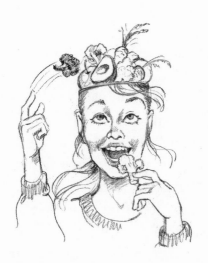

A healthy diet during the recovery from a brain injury is highly beneficial. Scientists know that deficiencies in certain nutrients and chemicals can cause disruptions in brain functioning and the ability to think clearly. The brain uses calories to function. When someone sustains a brain injury, it is necessary to eat enough nutritional calories to help the brain function efficiently.

Nutritional Tips for Head Injuries

- Eat small meals every three to four hours.
- Keep small baggies of healthy snacks with you during the day to boost your energy, such as nuts, trail mix, apples, cheese, hard-boiled eggs, and energy bars. Ask a member of your family or support group to make these for you and put them in a small cooler to take with you when away from home.
- Balance small meals with a combination of protein, healthy fats and oils, and carbohydrates. Proteins include fish, lean meats, nuts, and eggs. Healthy fats and oils can be found in avocados, seeds, and nuts. Carbohydrates are found in vegetables, fresh fruits, and grains. Avoid eating carbohydrates by themselves if you have blood sugar concerns. Many individuals report that sugar and chocolate increase headaches, so eat sweets sparingly.
- Eat moderately. Do not overeat as it can cause you to feel sleepy.
- Eat by the clock. If your brain/body signals are not working well, set a timer, watch alarm or a mobile phone to alert you that it's time to eat.

- Since weight gain is common following brain injury, this is another reason to stick to a healthy diet.
- Try to eat around the same time every day. The body does best when it is on a routine schedule.

Grocery Shopping and Menu Ideas

Shopping and preparing meals take a lot of energy. The grocery store is a very difficult environment when you have a head injury because of the lights, visual stimulation, and sounds.

- A magnetized notepad posted on the refrigerator is a time saver for writing down the food items to get during your next shopping trip. Photocopy a shopping list that you use regularly and circle the items you need to purchase during your next shopping trip. If you go to the same store each week, plan your list to follow the order of the aisles. For example, fresh foods usually line the walls or periphery of the grocery store, with packaged, canned, and frozen foods in the center aisles. This will help you conserve energy so that you won't have to make trips back and forth across the store.

- If you must go to the grocery store, try to choose a time when it is less crowded and less noisy. In the beginning, enlist the help of neighbors or friends to pick up the items on your shopping list when they are making a trip to the grocery store.
- If you are sensitive to noise and light, wear earplugs or filters and/or tinted glasses when shopping.
- Shop when you are well fed. You will make smarter food choices when you are not starving and your focus and attention will be sharper.
- Develop a list of your favorite fast, easy meal ideas. Keep this posted on your refrigerator or inside a cupboard door for easy access.
- Keep menus simple—avoid recipes with elaborate steps or unusual ingredients that aren't familiar to you.
- When preparing meals, always make extra to store in the refrigerator for the next day or two, or to put in the freezer. Put portions of foods into plastic or glass containers, and cover them with lids or plastic wrap.
- Throw protein foods out after three days in the refrigerator. Always practice safe food handling. Visit http://www.foodsafety.gov for further information.

- After a brain injury some people lose their sense of smell, and it is very important to be alert to the expiration dates on food.

What About Vitamins and Supplements?

There are many books and articles in magazines and on the Internet with tips and ideas for a healthy diet. It is highly recommended that fresh vegetables, fruits, fish, meats and grains are superior to processed foods and build the immune system. In addition, the following list of suggested supplements may help complement and enhance your nutritional intake.

- Multivitamins can supply the basic vitamins and supplements that your diet may be lacking.
- Omega-3 fatty acids counteract free radicals that cause oxidative damage to brain cells and may help improve nerve signal transmission at synapses.
- Probiotics is a beneficial bacteria that helps maintain a healthy intestine and aides in digestion.
- Antioxidants which include vitamins C, E, and beta carotene counteract oxidative damage caused by certain foods, and the stress caused by brain injury.
- Brain Vitale is a product that combines two beneficial brain nutrients which help repair

neurons—phosphatidyl serine and acetyl carnitine.

- Coenzyme Q10 is a natural antioxidant that is necessary for the basic functioning of cells.
- Phosphatidyl serine (PS) aids in the proper release and reception of neurotransmitters in the brain and helps with memory.
- Acetyl L-carnitine plays a key role in fatty acid oxidation and is used to improve memory.
- B vitamins boost metabolism and effect brain and nervous system functioning.
- GPC—glycerophosphocholine helps to sharpen alertness, reasoning, information processing, and other types of mental performance.

Consult a nutritionist or health care provider for an individualized program of supplementation. By eating well, you are developing a good foundation for recovery of your body and brain.

Foods to Avoid

Try to avoid the following foods:

- Alcohol
- Caffeine
- Salty foods
- Excessive sweets and candy

Warning:

You may find that if you drink alcohol following your injury, it may have a stronger effect than before because your tolerance level has changed. Alcohol may interact with prescription medications. Some people may turn to alcohol or other addictive substances to medicate themselves for physical or emotional pain. "It has been said that there should be no bottom line here. The use of these drugs in an already disrupted physiological system will further induce neurological and cognitive decline. They should be avoided by survivors of TBI."[1]

A little brain exercise daily goes a long way toward recovery. Cognitive exercise stimulates brain functioning just as aerobic exercise builds muscle.

CHAPTER 11

How to Improve Memory and Thinking Skills

Who Can Test and Treat Brain Functions?

Cognitive therapists and/or neuropsychologists can test brain functioning to assess the areas of strength and weakness. Neuropsychological testing is highly advanced and evaluates both the emotional and cognitive factors related to brain injury. Cognitive therapists, who treat brain injuries, are usually speech/language pathologists or occupational therapists who specialize in traumatic brain injury. They provide exercises to help strengthen brain functions, such as attention and concentration, memory, logical reasoning, problem solving, speed of processing, initiating activities, reading and math skills.

Some of the exercises use pencil and paper and some use software on the computer. Search the Internet for brain fitness websites to improve memory and cognitive skills. Refer to the list of resources in the back of the book for recommended websites. You also can purchase books that contain cognitive exercises at your local book store.

It is good to exercise your brain; however, it is important not to do exercises for long periods of time in the beginning, as this may overload your brain and cause an increase in your symptoms. Start with a maximum of five to ten minutes of brain exercises, until you know your brain's tolerance. Many times throughout this book, you will notice that we recommend a timer. It is an excellent way to remind you when to take a break.

If you start to get a headache or you have the sensation that your brain feels full, stop the task and consider putting an ice pack on the back of your neck. Also, if there are brain-related activities that you find difficult in the beginning, your cognitive therapist can suggest ways for you to compensate until your brain is ready to advance.

Brain Stretchers

A little brain exercise daily goes a long way toward recovery. Cognitive exercise stimulates brain functioning just as aerobic exercise builds muscle.

When you are able to think without tiring, the following activities can help the brain form new information pathways and perform more efficiently. Your providers will have additional suggestions.

Crossword puzzles give your word-finding skills a workout. Frequently, word retrieval skills are affected by the injury, and remembering even simple words can be tough. You will quickly graduate to more challenging levels. Take breaks and consider finishing a difficult crossword puzzle the next day. You will be surprised how quickly the answers show up after you have rested or have had a good night's sleep.

Cognitive therapists can provide specific rehabilitation programs to improve brain functioning. You will find a list of cognitive therapists on www.asha.org.

Watching the Wheel of Fortune on TV can be an entertaining way of exercising your recall skills. There are programs available on the Internet designed to improve cognition, speed of processing, and memory skills. For recommended web sites, go to www.Lumosity.com, www. puzzlersparadise.com, www.CogniFit.com, and www. braingle.com. Many people also find the Nintendo DS Lite with Brain Age software to be convenient and portable.

Sudoku puzzles are an excellent way to work on sequencing, planning, and problem solving. These are great exercises because you can stop at any time and then pick them up later without losing your place. Start with the easy level and build up to the more challenging levels.

Logic puzzles help to break down the thinking process into smaller steps. The rapid speed at which your brain used to come to conclusions may have been affected, and trying to make those "snap" decisions now can be difficult. Logic puzzles use reasoning and brain focus to draw conclusions.

Card games and board games provide social opportunities for laughter and companionship. Some games to consider include Scrabble, Scattergories, Taboo, and Rush Hour. Card games such as Crazy Eights, Gin Rummy, and Bridge are excellent for sharpening the brain. Also consider Solitaire, but use playing cards rather than the computer, as it exercises your logic and eye-hand coordination.

What Does Exercise Have To Do with It?

Physical exercise is an important part of recovery from a brain injury, even if it's walking a short distance a few times a week. Be sure to consult your doctor and/or physical therapist before returning to physical exercise. In the early stages of recovery, be cautious when engaging in physical activities where the brain may be jarred, for example running, horseback riding, skiing, mountain biking and motocross. It is also important to assess whether you can process information and react as quickly as you could previously. In activities that require rapid reaction times, it may be difficult to meet the physical challenges until your reaction time improves.

We all know that physical exercise makes us feel better because it alleviates stress and increases the flow of endorphins. Dr. Ratey, author of *Spark: The Revolutionary New Science of Exercise and the Brain,* states that "physical exercise can sharpen your thinking, improve memory skills, and prepare the brain for learning." He also talks about the many scientifically proven benefits of aerobic exercise and emphasizes the relationship of exercise and mood elevation.[1]

Current research on exercise and brain functioning reveals the following:

- Aerobic exercise increases blood flow to the brain.
- Exercise increases the level of brain-derived neurotropic factor (BDNF), which is like brain fertilizer and can help with integrity of neurons and other neuronal structures.
- Exercise enhances mood, most likely due to the release of endorphins.

Biofeedback has been shown to decrease anxiety responses and may allow you to go into a relaxation response rather than a stress response.

CHAPTER 12

What Is Biofeedback and Neurofeedback?

Biofeedback and EEG neurofeedback have been documented as successful treatment modalities for MTBI.[1] EEG biofeedback has been shown as an effective intervention for treating auditory memory problems in TBI.[2] And quantitative EEG is a highly sensitive diagnostic tool in identifying post concussion syndrome.[3] Currently, there are numerous biofeedback and neurofeedback training programs for optimal performance that have shown good preliminary results in reducing or eliminating symptoms of TBI and PTSD.[4] Biofeedback/neurofeedback was also studied by Dr. Eugene Peniston for the treatment of combat-related, post traumatic stress disorder and substance abuse.[5]

Biofeedback is the use of sensitive instruments to measure physical responses in the body and feed them back to you in order to help alter your body's responses. You can observe the feedback on a computer screen or listen to sound feedback.

Biofeedback Treatment Options

Different types of biofeedback are used to treat various physical and emotional problems. For example:

- Electromyographic (EMG) biofeedback may be used to treat muscle tension headaches as well as neck pain, jaw pain, etc.
- Temperature biofeedback helps you learn to increase blood flow into various parts of the body. Having a head injury may cause temperature dysregulation. Many individuals report feeling very hot or very cold.
- Electrodermal response (EDR) is a way to measure the body's tendency to go into a fight-or-flight response. This may happen after a traumatic event.
- Pneumographic biofeedback (breathing biofeedback) is a modality used to measure chest versus abdominal breathing. This can help you learn to breathe more deeply and regularly to improve your relaxation response.

- Heart rate variability biofeedback brings the
cardiovascular and physiological systems
into harmony, which may positively affect
conditions, such as depression and anxiety.
- EEG neurofeedback or brain-wave biofeedback
is a form of biofeedback in which surface
electrodes are placed on the scalp to measure
specific brain-wave frequencies and provide
feedback to the individual. You may learn
to suppress or enhance specific brain-wave
frequencies, thus enabling you to learn to focus,
relax, and increase flexibility of thinking.
- The primary brain-wave frequencies that are
measured include delta, theta, alpha, low beta,
and beta. Different brain-wave frequencies are
associated with various states and various
disorders. For example, individuals with
traumatic brain injuries frequently have an
abundance of theta waves, or low-frequency
brain waves. Attention deficit disorders also
reveal high levels of theta. The goal of this
treatment is to teach individuals to move
flexibly in and out of certain brain-wave
states to enhance performance. If theta levels
are too high and you cannot focus, you may
want to learn to suppress that wave and
increase alpha and beta which will allow

you to be more focused and present. Many of the neurofeedback protocols used with TBI and PTSD also involve sensorimotor rhythm (SMR) training.

Treatment Techniques

In conjunction with visual and auditory feedback from the biofeedback equipment and brain-wave machines, individuals are encouraged to practice daily techniques to enhance their skill levels.

Following are some of the most successful techniques:

- Progressive muscle relaxation
- Deep muscle relaxation
- Breathing and muscle awareness
- Autogenic relaxation or rapid relaxation
- Visual imagery
- Open-focus training
- Systematic desensitization, a technique that helps develop an internal sense of control
- Short relaxation forms (e.g., quieting response, body stress scanning)
- Carryover techniques to bring the strategies into everyday life

Benefits Gained from Biofeedback and Neurofeedback

The benefits of biofeedback depend on the skills you want to learn. For example, you may learn to warm your hands, which may, in turn, lower your blood pressure or decrease migraine headaches. By learning to relax the muscles in your face, neck, shoulders, and back, you may be able to eliminate or decrease tension headaches, jaw pain, back pain, or clenching and grinding of your teeth. By learning to go into a relaxation response rather than a stress response, you can decrease anxiety.

The benefits of neurofeedback are many. For example, you may learn to alter your brain-wave frequencies to decrease foggy thinking and increase clarity and cognitive stamina. It is important to see a provider who is certified by the Biofeedback Certification International Alliance (www.bcia.org).

Give yourself all the time you need to heal.
Avoid putting yourself on a timetable.
Your recovery is a major life transformation.

CHAPTER 13

Redefining Recovery

Where is the magic wand when we need it? Recovery time varies from person to person, although it is never as fast as we would like it to be. To some people with a brain injury, the word "recovery" means regaining what you lost, the pain goes away and the brain is as sharp and attentive as it was before the accident. However, every brain injury is as varied as the recovery process because of the uniqueness of who you are. A brain injury is unlike all other injuries.

When injured, the brain shuts down to protect itself. As the recovery process continues, the brain wakes up and the fog lifts. If you haven't started the rehabilitation process, it is now time for the gentle help of cognitive, physical and emotional rehabilitation. There are many articles and books about people who have made miraculous recoveries from head injuries and gone on to thrive and live happy and productive lives.

In fact, some individuals actually report that they are better than they were prior to the injury because they now understand the brain and what it needs to thrive. They have learned how to stimulate brain functioning, how to exercise their bodies efficiently, how to judge the amount of sleep they need, and how to feed their bodies nutritionally to help them maintain healthy lifestyles.

Redefining recovery from MTBI is about growing and changing. The cells of the body are constantly being replaced according to their own schedule and demand. As we mature, we may change our beliefs, attitudes and life strategies which are influenced by experiences, relationships, and current situations. We may change our preferences for foods, music, leisure activities or where we want to live, whether it is near cities, mountains, plains or oceans. We may even change the kinds of people we want as friends.

Certain events in our lives can change the course or direction you thought you were going. Recovery is not only about regaining what you lost, it is also about adjusting to the change and reinventing yourself on many levels. In the process of this transformation your perspective of the world and of yourself may change. It is a state of mind, as they say, or a state of being your true self. It is a place where you can make sense of the world and trust your gut feelings and your intuition. In order to achieve this state of being, it requires you to slow your life down and become more conscious—more aware. This allows time for introspection, to gain insight and the ability to make confident decisions and wise choices.

When you are feeling stronger, find ways to immerse yourself creatively through music, art, writing, reading, hobbies, etc. In your newfound gratefulness you may be inspired to find ways to give back to those caring people who have helped you along the way.

As you heal and start to reach out and interact more, there may be a desire to bring meaning, purpose, and a sense of belonging back into your life. There may be new opportunities to be part of a group, a place where you feel validated and can share joy and laughter. Perhaps it is with your friends and co-workers, in your career, family, community, church, or in nature.

No Time Limits

Give yourself all the time you need to heal. Avoid putting yourself on a timetable. Your recovery is a major life transformation. Be prepared to change your life to work with your injury, not against it. Give yourself double the amount of time you would have previously given yourself to complete a task.

It may be wise to delay going back to work on a full-time basis. Give your brain time to recover. If there is anything you take away from this book, please let it be this: slow down and pace yourself.

Stair-step Recovery Model

Although many individuals recover from MTBI within the first 90 days, the initial healing time is typically 18-24 months. Many say that they still notice recovery between three to five years post-injury. The first 90 days is called the period of "rapid spontaneous recovery," when the brain is going through spontaneous healing.

Brain injuries recover in what is known as stair-step recovery which is illustrated in Figure 2.

Figure 2. Stair-Step Recovery Model

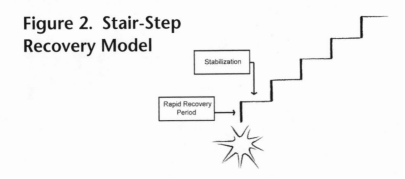

Recovery moves through a series of steps where you will most likely notice a rapid recovery period followed by a stabilization period. This pattern repeats itself over time. When you are in the stabilization or "flat" part of the stair step, you may think that you will stay as you are and not continue to recover.

The majority of individuals find, however, that they continue to see improvements across many areas of cognitive functioning over many years. This is a positive aspect of the recovery process. By understanding the stair-step recovery model, it gives you the realistic hope you need over time to stay with the healing process.

Comments We've All Heard

One of the most frustrating aspects of having MTBI is that there is no apparent wound or readily visible sign of your injury. People will tell you how good you look, how you don't seem injured, or encourage you to believe that you are healed before you are. Please understand that they mean well and are trying to make you feel better.

Here are some comments we've all heard:

- "You look fine."
- "You don't look sick."
- "Oh, that happens to me all the time."
- "That's just part of getting older."

- "So, just get a different job."
- "How much longer does this go on?"
- "You're still seeing doctors!?"
- "It could have been worse."
- "Just snap out of it."

It Is What It Is!

Accept the fact that you are injured, and treat yourself like you might treat an injured loved one—with lots of pampering and compassion. It's normal to have mood swings and feel adrift. Remain flexible. It is what it is! You will know when the time is right to go to the next level of activity and thinking.

If you are taking good care of yourself, you are fitting rest times into your busy schedule. Meditation, biofeedback, and breathing exercises can all be extremely helpful.

A typical breathing exercise is to breathe in to the count of four and breathe out to the count of eight. Repeat eight to ten times. Breathing exercises have been known to calm the anxious mind and lower blood pressure.

Visualization is another way to quiet your brain and help your body to relax. Use your own memory tapes to recall happy occasions. Use positive images to redirect your thinking. Music is also a powerful mood changer. The companionship of a pet has been shown to be "good medicine." Various organizations, such as, Freedom Dogs, are enlisting canines to assist people with MTBI and PTSD. They also assist troops at home and abroad. Check out the following web site: www.freedomdogs.org.

Try It, You Might Like It

Success stories happen every day with this type of injury. People who have never even thought of writing, have written and published books after their injury. Some have pursued careers in the arts, and others have explored new occupations through vocational rehabilitation. You may discover talents that you never knew you had.

Did you ever think of learning to play that musical instrument you always wanted to try, but put aside the dream for more practical pursuits? Many of these creative activities integrate both sides of the brain and promote healing in a more profound way.

Creating Support Systems

It is important to talk with people who understand what you are going through. Doctors and therapists trained in the symptoms and treatment of MTBI will be supportive and understanding. You may also need family or couple's counseling to help your significant other understand your feelings about this radical change in your life. Therapy also gives them a chance to discuss their concerns and confusion.

Try to find a brain injury support group in your area. Ask your therapist or healthcare providers if they know of any. Contact your state Brain Injury Association, or the National Brain Injury Association at 1-800-444-6443, or at www.biausa.org, for more information. Refer to the "Resources" section in the back of this book for an expanded list.

Services are available to help you with the day-to-day chores that can become overwhelming. Some grocery stores offer shopping and delivery service. Your friends may be willing to run errands, cook meals, make phone calls, and even car pool the kids around.

And finally, rather than focusing on your disabilities, focus on your abilities. When you shift your attention, you will be surprised to find new skills that you have acquired during this transformational time. Take a moment now and honestly ask yourself, "What's new and different about me that I like?" "What's new and different about me that other people like?"

Remember to delegate—simplify—dump!

My Thoughts and Observations

If this is an automobile accident, regardless of how minor the accident is, always call the police to the scene of the accident or ask someone to call for you.

CHAPTER 14

What Are My Insurance and Legal Rights?

It is amazing what we don't know about our insurance policies or our legal rights until an accident happens. Sometimes, we discover that our insurance policy does not have enough coverage and most learning is done in hindsight. Whether you are reading this chapter before, in the middle of, or after an accident, hopefully, the following information will make you a more informed insurance policy owner.

Getting Organized

In order to eliminate confusion, create an "Accident File" for all pertinent information regarding the accident, whether it was caused by an automobile accident, fall, sports-related injury or on the job. Keep separate folders for each provider with insurance statements and corresponding provider billing statements, as well as, therapy appointments, lab test results, medical appointments, and medications. Perhaps a friend or family member can help you maintain these files. Be sure to pick up business cards from each new medical provider you see and keep them together for future reference. List them in an address book, on the computer, or in the appropriate medical provider files. Some people have taped the business cards to a piece of paper to keep them readily available all in one place.

Insurance Questions To Consider

Inform your insurance company immediately. Since insurance benefits vary from state to state regarding type of coverage, policy guarantees and medical coverage, the following questions will help you become better informed:

- Do I need to have pre-authorization for treatment?
- Can I choose my own providers?
- What are the policy limits on medical and rehabilitation treatments?
- Is there a time limit during which treatment can be obtained?
- Does the policy cover mileage expenses to providers?

- Does the policy cover taxi fares, if I am unable to drive?
- Does the policy cover lost wages for time off from work?
- Are essential services covered, such as cleaning, cooking, shopping, driving, etc.?
- How do you define essential services?
- Is there anything else you feel I should know?

If this is a work-related injury, try to notify your employer first, so that the accident can be documented and the appropriate paperwork completed. If possible, ask your employer the name of the designated doctor, clinic or emergency room to go to for an evaluation and/or treatment. Getting the care you need is the most important thing. In workers' compensation claims you usually have a primary occupational medicine doctor who supervises your case and prescribes treatments, medications, and coordinates your care with other providers.

If this is an automobile accident, regardless of how minor the accident, always call the police to the scene of the accident or ask someone to call for you. If police were not called, it is important to file a police report immediately after the accident. Even if there are no obvious wounds, go to the emergency room and be assessed by a medical professional and be sure to tell them all of your symptoms.

They may want to take x-rays, and/or brain imaging studies, if appropriate.

When you file an auto insurance claim, an insurance adjustor will contact you for your report of the accident. Hopefully, at the time of the accident you or someone else had the presence of mind to take photos of your car and the other vehicle/s involved at the scene of the accident. Get the names of witnesses at the accident scene. You are entitled to a copy of the police report of the accident. Be sure to verify that the facts are accurate, for example, the names of drivers involved, who the ticket was issued to, the speed of the vehicles, names and contact information for witnesses, and the location of the accident.

When you are asked to give a report of the accident for insurance purposes, be honest and clear and do not minimize what happened to you, since it is important to document all of the details of the accident. Your initial description of the accident will often be tape recorded. Keeping a journal is extremely helpful in these situations. Do not sign a waiver, or accept a quick settlement.

Don't delay your treatment, and be sure to get all the necessary treatment as soon as possible. If you have an attorney, ask for specific guidelines on how to best communicate with your insurance company from the very beginning. The auto insurance company may cover some treatment expenses while the health insurance company may cover others. They will sort out the costs when the claim settles. In some situations, disability insurance or Social Security Disability Income (SSDI) may also be available.

Some insurance companies may be helpful, but others may delay or deny payment for hospital or medical services. That is why it is critical to stay alert regarding your bills. By asking questions regarding why a payment is denied, you may discover that the insurance company does not have all the documents necessary to process your claim. If you cannot get satisfaction, ask your attorney to act as your go-between. Keep copies of all correspondence and claims and be sure to consult your attorney before giving any statements to your insurance company.

Since insurance companies have a language all their own, try to get familiar with the many new terms. For example, most policies will cover treatment that is "reasonable" and "medically necessary" for your recovery. Always ask questions if you do not understand their procedures or if the explanations seem confusing.

In some states you must buy medical pay at the time you buy your policy to cover the cost of accident-related medical bills. Additionally, it may be important to have uninsured motorist/underinsured motorist coverage as part of your policy.

You may have financial challenges if your policy coverage is exhausted and you are still unable to return to work. If you have creditors, explain the situation and ask for assistance in paying your debt, or set up a payment plan to avoid being turned over to collections. If you have an attorney, this may be an area to ask for clarification.

Do I Need an Attorney?

You may need the help of a qualified attorney who handles personal injury or workers' compensation cases, and who deals with and understands MTBI. It is important to ask the right questions when selecting an attorney because you will be working very closely with this person, and you want to have trust in their skills and approach. Your doctors, therapists or other people with MTBI may be able to suggest some names of competent attorneys to start the process of finding someone who is right for you. Some important questions include:

- Have you represented other individuals with MTBI in personal injury cases? What has the outcome been?

- Do you work closely with medical professionals, rehabilitation specialists, vocational rehabilitation experts, and economists who calculate lost income?
- Do you understand the subtleties of MTBI (e.g. visual problems, cognitive problems, hypersensitivity to sound and light, etc.)?

Once you determine the questions that are important to you, then interview several attorneys and choose one who makes you feel comfortable. You may want to take someone with you during the interview process. Keep in mind that there are time-sensitive issues in legal cases and you must pay attention to deadlines. An attorney can help keep track of these deadlines.

What About Legal Fees?

Most attorneys will not charge you until the case is settled in personal injury cases. This is called a contingency fee. At settlement they usually charge a percentage, plus any expenses they incur, in the course of handling your case. If cases go to court, the attorney's fees and the percentage they take may increase because of the additional resources, time and work that is required. Be sure to ask the exact percentage you are being charged because it can vary depending on whether your case goes to court. In addition to the contingency fee, you are usually responsible for the direct costs to the attorney, but this should be included in your contract.

Your attorney can advise you of your legal rights, file all necessary paperwork, and look out for your best interests. Attorneys can help take the stress out of dealing with insurance companies, and they frequently get better results from insurance companies than you would if you tried to deal with them directly. Once you hire an attorney, that person will talk with your insurance adjustor and help deal with insurance-related issues.

Your attorney will help get your medical bills paid and recover any damages for you. Oftentimes, your attorney will assign a paralegal professional to handle your case on a day-to-day basis. However, if you need to speak directly with the attorney, they should be willing to do so. It may be necessary to set up an appointment to speak to your attorney in person to ensure that you understand important deadlines and discuss important aspects of your case. You have the right to change attorneys at any time during your case, if you are dissatisfied with the management of your case.

Keep a file of your medical records, insurance claims, and conversations with whom you speak to about your case, as this may be helpful. Note the date and write down the names of all contacts. Maneuvering through the insurance and legal system can be difficult especially if this is a new experience for you.

The Independent Medical Exam (IME)

An IME is an Independent Medical Examination, which is performed by an Independent Medical Examiner chosen by the insurance company to evaluate your condition and treatment, and to determine whether it is reasonable and medically necessary. An insurance company may choose to set up an appointment for you at any point in time during the recovery process; however, the exam is typically scheduled six months to one year after your treatment begins. A neurologist, physiatrist, psychologist, or other doctor or therapist may perform the IME.

When you see an examiner, be very clear about which treatments have helped you. Ask someone to go with you to the exam and take notes. This person may or may not be allowed into the examination room. It is your right to ask the examiner how much experience they have with MTBI patients.

You should have the right to see the examiner's written report to the insurance company. If you disagree with the findings, you have the right to challenge them by writing a rebuttal letter. It is best to consult your attorney on these rights. Also, your attorney and healthcare providers can write letters of rebuttal if the IME report recommends that treatment be discontinued.

Please note that the IME procedure can vary from state to state. For this reason having an attorney represent you is so very important. Remember that you are legally entitled to all reasonable and necessary treatment for the length of time, or the dollar amount stated in the insurance policy.

My Thoughts and Observations

*You have just taken a detour on your life's journey.
There is so much more to experience and discover
if you are open to the endless possibilities.*

CHAPTER 15

Hey, Do I Get My Old Life Back?

Many of us ask, "When can I return to work?" or, "When can I do the things that I used to do?" The honest answer is . . . "who knows?" You may find that you don't want your old life back. Maybe the stress and confusion of your old life are no longer desirable, or maybe you just aren't able to do what you used to do before the injury.

You have just taken a detour on your life's journey. There is so much more to experience and discover, if you are open to the endless possibilities. Try new things but respect your new limitations. Remember not to force yourself. Discover what you enjoy doing now. Really, when you think about it, we are all growing and changing in many ways.

The core essence of who you are will never change; it is how you choose to express it from now on. You have just experienced a significant, life-changing event. It is your choice if you will be the victim or the victor, and in the early stages of recovery, you may play both of these roles. Months or even years later, as you look back, you will be amazed at how far you have come in your recovery and in reinventing yourself.

Perhaps, you might view it as a second chance or the beginning of the next chapter in your life. Use this transition in a positive way. This will be one of the greatest challenges you will ever face and some of the greatest gifts that you will ever receive.

It is exciting to learn, as the latest research confirms, that we all have magnificent brains. In the next chapter, you will be encouraged by the landmark studies that reveal how the brain has the ability to heal and change in ways you never imagined.

It's Not About You

When we have a life-altering event such as a brain injury, it is natural to take things more personally. It may seem that friends, work associates, and even loved ones do not understand. If they have not experienced a head injury, they may not have an understanding of what you are going through. No one can possibly know your personal journey in this recovery process. Let them know what you are experiencing so that they can assist you.

It is difficult not to take things personally, particularly when you are overloaded, fatigued, and in pain. This may be a first-time experience for everyone involved. It's not just about you—it's about all of us developing understanding and compassion for this life-changing event.

Seek out organizations that give advice, assistance, and treatment, such as local brain injury associations. Join support groups, share experiences, and learn from others. Don't forget to share the humorous incidents because laughter is a powerful healer.

The human brain is an amazing and flexible organ. This is one of the many reasons why the brain can be rehabilitated following an injury.

CHAPTER 16

What's the Good News?

The Amazing Brain

The human brain is an amazing and flexible organ. It weighs about three pounds and contains approximately 100 billion nerve cells.[1] It is believed that the 100 billion neurons in the brain are able to talk with each other through one or more links. Once a linkage is formed, it becomes stronger through repetition. This is one of the many reasons why the brain can be rehabilitated and retrained after it is injured.

Dr. Eric Braverman, in his book, *The Edge Effect*, states that the difference between a brain that is resourceful and functioning well and one that isn't, is only 100 milliseconds of brain speed.[2] As the brain ages or becomes injured in an accident, it may process information more slowly. However, with practice and determination and by working to improve memory, speed of processing and focused concentration, you can overcome what you think is holding you back. At the same time, you may learn strategies to compensate. Some skills may be taken away or diminished, but you may also gain new skills that you never thought were possible.

What Is Brain Neuroplasticity?

Neuroplasticity is the brain's ability to change itself. The good news is that the brain is resilient and trainable. It is believed that the brain can open old pathways, regenerate new pathways, and may even grow new brain cells to help it function normally again. Treatment to help the brain regain skills is called cognitive retraining.

The brain has a left and right hemisphere and four major lobes—frontal, parietal, temporal, and occipital. The corpus callosum connects the two hemispheres of the brain with interconnecting fibers. The left hemisphere oversees linear functions and language, mathematical computation, reading, verbal memory, word recall, etc. The right hemisphere has to do with such things as nonlinear, creative thinking, humor, simple math computation, musical talents, etc. The Frontal Lobe is very important in brain injury and controls reasoning, problem solving, and planning. The Parietal Lobe assists with orientation and sensory stimuli. The Occipital Lobe regulates visual reception and processing; and the Temporal Lobe controls auditory reception and language. Please refer to Figure 3.

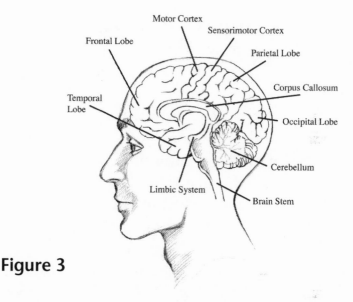

Figure 3

Recent research and the progress of brain imaging studies are highlighting the fact that many functions occur in multiple areas of the brain. Through these sensitive diagnostic tools, brain functions will be more clearly identified.

The good news is that the brain is highly resilient. This means that it can compensate for problems and it can be rehabilitated to perform more normally again, even following an injury. The brain has the ability to change with brain fitness exercises. If you would like to learn more about the magnificent brain, we highly recommend the book, *The Brain That Changes Itself,* by Norman Doidge, MD.[3]

It is important to talk with your doctor before initiating a program. The brain needs to rest initially following an injury before it begins retraining exercises. When you start exercising the brain, perform tasks for very brief periods of time (five to ten minutes). Discovering your tolerance level will allow you and your therapist to design a program that fits the specific amount of time and the type of tasks that you can perform.

Change your activity by going for a walk, do breathing exercises, or dance to music. Do whatever it takes to increase the blood flow to give your brain a boost in oxygen in a gentle way, especially in the beginning. You will be surprised how a ten or fifteen-minute break can sharpen your thinking. You may need to rest and close your eyes for a period of time to recharge the brain, then go back to the project or activity for brief periods, followed by relaxing and recharging breaks. Alternating brain rest and stimulation is called "pacing." This is a very important activity to accelerate brain recovery.

When you are ready, here are some tips for TRAINING your brain:

1. Focus on new learning—play a musical instrument, learn to speak a new language, try new or novel tasks and activities.
2. Start your brain training with tasks that you can accomplish without significant effort.
3. Use the idea of REVERSALS—e.g., use your left hand versus your right hand, perform visual versus auditory tasks, etc.
4. Engage in tasks that encourage the brain to become flexible in its thinking patterns (e.g., say patterns like AB 1, 2; CD 3, 4; EF 5, 6, etc).
5. Stimulate the brain by listening to music and try to recall the words. Read articles and try to recall one or two things that you read. Then, try to recall them an hour later.
6. Refer to the "Resources" section for suggested reading. Try not to get discouraged, especially if you find it hard in the beginning to concentrate or focus. A trained cognitive therapist will help you design a cognitive program that will improve your brain function at a pace that is best for you.

The Path of Mystery

One of the great mysteries in life is "WHY" something happens. Why did I sustain an injury? Why am I in so much pain? Why is my loved one suffering so much? Unfortunately, we frequently do not get to know why something happens. We only know that we have a new opportunity in life to respond in a way that will advance our healing and strengthen our internal life force.

For those who have faith, this type of injury can be a call to faith. For those who don't, this can be a beckoning to something much bigger.

We did a little study over time with our clients who had suffered brain injuries. When they had completed their treatment, they were asked why they believed they had sustained this type of injury and, if given the choice, would they move along this path and take this same journey again. Without exception, they said, "yes," they would, by choice, have the injury because it was a rich life experience. The majority of the individuals believed that it opened a door to a spiritual journey for them.

The mystery of life comes in many forms. Your nature will be tested and your true strengths will shine through. It is sometimes difficult to see the gifts of such a long and demanding journey with so little relief. Many believe that it builds patience and endurance, and others talk about the ability to find compassion for others through their own suffering.

Some individuals talk about learning to forgive another person or a situation. It is truly an opportunity to question all of your previous beliefs and listen to a deeper calling. Some believe that, when the whisper doesn't get your attention, you may be awakened by something more profound—like a brain injury, a physical loss, or an emotional trauma.

Although the road has many twists and turns, the learning experience is unique. It takes a great deal of strength and courage to believe that you will recover, and to shed the bitterness and anger that you may feel for what may appear to be senseless suffering. By taking care of yourself and following a path of recovery, you give everyone hope. It is a precious gift to allow others to help you. Aspire to find hope and love in those around you. You are not alone.

Medical Definition of MTBI

The Mild Traumatic Brain Injury Committee of the Head Injury Interdisciplinary Special Interest Group of the American Congress of Rehabilitation Medicine published the following, which is a more specific medical definition of MTBI (1993):

A patient with mild traumatic brain injury is a person who has had a traumatically-induced physiological disruption of brain function, as manifested by at least one of the following:

1. Any period or loss of consciousness
2. Any loss of memory for events immediately before or after the accident
3. Any alteration in mental state at the time of the accident—feeling dazed, disoriented, or confused
4. Focal neurological deficit(s) that may or may not be transient, but where the severity of the injury does not exceed the following:

- Post-traumatic amnesia (PTA) not greater than twenty-four hours
- After thirty minutes, an initial Glasgow Coma Scale (GCS) of 13 to 15*
- Loss of consciousness of approximately thirty minutes or less

*Glasgow Coma Scale (GCS) is a neurological scale with a 1 to 15-point scoring system that is used to record levels of consciousness. It assesses best eye response, best verbal response, and best motor response. The lowest GCS score possible is a sum of 3; and the highest is 15, "fully awake."

Functional Symptom Questionnaire

The following questionnaire (which begins on the next page) was designed to evaluate many areas of cognitive functioning based on the perceptions of the individual. It is used to measure progress over time. It is a valid and reliable tool used to discriminate between mild to moderate TBI and non-injured individuals. It is suggested that you retake this Functional Symptom Questionnaire every three to six months to measure your progress.

Functional Symptom Questionnaire

Name: _____

Date: _____

Please read this list (or have it read to you) and indicate any problems that you may be experiencing. Rate your problems on this scale: Almost Never, Occasionally, Sometimes, Frequently, Almost Always. Circle the category that best matches your response.

Memory

1. Are you losing or misplacing items?

Almost Never | Occasionally | Sometimes | Frequently | Almost Always

2. Are you forgetting what people tell you?

Almost Never | Occasionally | Sometimes | Frequently | Almost Always

3. Do you forget where you parked your car?

Almost Never | Occasionally | Sometimes | Frequently | Almost Always

4. Are you forgetting what you've read?

Almost Never | Occasionally | Sometimes | Frequently | Almost Always

5. Are you having difficulty remembering things from the past?

Almost Never | Occasionally | Sometimes | Frequently | Almost Always

Attention and Concentration

1. Are you having trouble concentrating?

Almost Never | Occasionally | Sometimes | Frequently | Almost Always

2. Do you have difficulty concentrating in noisy environments?

Almost Never | Occasionally | Sometimes | Frequently | Almost Always

3. Do you have difficulty concentrating on more than one thing at a time?

Almost Never | Occasionally | Sometimes | Frequently | Almost Always

4. Do you have difficulty focusing your attention while reading or watching TV?

Almost Never | Occasionally | Sometimes | Frequently | Almost Always

5. Are you having difficulty staying focused when you are driving?

Almost Never | Occasionally | Sometimes | Frequently | Almost Always

Language and Communication

1. Do you have difficulty understanding other people or following a conversation?

Almost Never | Occasionally | Sometimes | Frequently | Almost Always

2. Do you have difficulty thinking of words?

Almost Never | Occasionally | Sometimes | Frequently | Almost Always

3. Do you have problems expressing yourself in writing?

Almost Never | Occasionally | Sometimes | Frequently | Almost Always

4. Do you have difficulty expressing yourself verbally (e.g., do people ask you to repeat yourself)?

Almost Never | Occasionally | Sometimes | Frequently | Almost Always

5. Do you have difficulty spelling words?

Almost Never | Occasionally | Sometimes | Frequently | Almost Always

Balance/Coordination/Sensory Function

1. Do you find you have difficulty with handwriting, hitting a ball, riding a bicycle, or doing something that used to be easy to do?

Almost Never | Occasionally | Sometimes | Frequently | Almost Always

2. Do you have problems with balance or coordination?

Almost Never | Occasionally | Sometimes | Frequently | Almost Always

3. Do you experience increased fatigability?

Almost Never | Occasionally | Sometimes | Frequently | Almost Always

4. Do you experience loss or decrease in sense of taste?

Almost Never | Occasionally | Sometimes | Frequently | Almost Always

5. Do you experience loss or decrease in sense of smell?

Almost Never | Occasionally | Sometimes | Frequently | Almost Always

6. Do you experience physical pain?

Almost Never | Occasionally | Sometimes | Frequently | Almost Always

7. Do you experience sleep disturbance?

Almost Never | Occasionally | Sometimes | Frequently | Almost Always

Visual-Perception

1. Do you have increased sensitivity to light?

Almost Never | Occasionally | Sometimes | Frequently | Almost Always

2. Do objects seem closer or farther away than they actually are?

Almost Never | Occasionally | Sometimes | Frequently | Almost Always

3. When reading, do printed letters appear to change or change position? Do you see two of things when there is only one?

Almost Never | Occasionally | Sometimes | Frequently | Almost Always

4. Do you have difficulty focusing your eyes on objects?

Almost Never | Occasionally | Sometimes | Frequently | Almost Always

5. Do you feel dizzy or nauseous?

Almost Never | Occasionally | Sometimes | Frequently | Almost Always

Executive Function

1. Do you have difficulty planning work or leisure activities?

Almost Never | Occasionally | Sometimes | Frequently | Almost Always

2. Do you have problems setting goals and priorities?

Almost Never | Occasionally | Sometimes | Frequently | Almost Always

3. Do you have difficulty starting new tasks?

Almost Never | Occasionally | Sometimes | Frequently | Almost Always

4. Do you have difficulty monitoring and correcting your errors?

Almost Never | Occasionally | Sometimes | Frequently | Almost Always

5. Do you have difficulty changing from one task to another?

Almost Never | Occasionally | Sometimes | Frequently | Almost Always

Emotional Functioning

1. Have you noticed increased moodiness?

Almost Never | Occasionally | Sometimes | Frequently | Almost Always

2. Do you lose your temper more quickly than before?

Almost Never | Occasionally | Sometimes | Frequently | Almost Always

3. Do you feel depressed?

Almost Never | Occasionally | Sometimes | Frequently | Almost Always

4. Do you have feelings of anxiety or nervousness?

Almost Never | Occasionally | Sometimes | Frequently | Almost Always

5. Do family and friends comment on changes in your behavior?

Almost Never | Occasionally | Sometimes | Frequently | Almost Always

6. Do you have increased irritability?

Almost Never | Occasionally | Sometimes | Frequently | Almost Always

Finances and Measurements

1. Do you have difficulty performing simple addition and subtraction?

Almost Never | Occasionally | Sometimes | Frequently | Almost Always

2. Do you have difficulty making change at the store?

Almost Never | Occasionally | Sometimes | Frequently | Almost Always

3. Do you have difficulty balancing your checkbook as accurately as before?

Almost Never | Occasionally | Sometimes | Frequently | Almost Always

4. Do you have difficulty paying your bills on time?

Almost Never | Occasionally | Sometimes | Frequently | Almost Always

5. Do you have difficulty calculating the appropriate measurements for receipes or other projects?

Almost Never | Occasionally | Sometimes | Frequently | Almost Always

Organization and Sequencing

1. Do you have difficulty following the steps of a recipe?

Almost Never | Occasionally | Sometimes | Frequently | Almost Always

2. Are you having difficulty attending to your mail on a regular basis?

Almost Never | Occasionally | Sometimes | Frequently | Almost Always

3. Are you having difficulty doing or keeping up with normal routine household chores?

Almost Never | Occasionally | Sometimes | Frequently | Almost Always

4. Do you have difficulty doing more than one thing at a time?

Almost Never | Occasionally | Sometimes | Frequently | Almost Always

5. Do you have difficulty effectively managing your time?

Almost Never | Occasionally | Sometimes | Frequently | Almost Always

Safety

1. Do you forget to turn off the iron, stove, or other electrical appliances?

Almost Never | Occasionally | Sometimes | Frequently | Almost Always

2. Do you forget where you're going when you get into your car?

Almost Never | Occasionally | Sometimes | Frequently | Almost Always

3. Do you forget to lock your doors at home?

Almost Never | Occasionally | Sometimes | Frequently | Almost Always

4. Do you forget important appointments (e.g., picking up your children, etc.)?

Almost Never | Occasionally | Sometimes | Frequently | Almost Always

5. Do you feel that your awareness levels are less than they should be?

Almost Never | Occasionally | Sometimes | Frequently | Almost Always

Understanding Your Results

There are 53 items on the Functional Symptom Questionnaire. By adding up the number of each response (Almost Never, Occasionally, Sometimes, Frequently, and Almost Always), and dividing each one by the total number of items in the questionnaire (53), you will get a percentage "of how often you have symptoms at each severity level. For example, if you have 10 in the Almost Always category and divide 10 by 53, your result will be 19%. This questionnaire was designed to measure your progress over time. Try using this assessment tool every three to six months to track your progress and to pinpoint areas that need attention. Remember, the healing process is unique to everyone and the physical, emotional, cognitive and thinking abilities improve at different rates.

Medication Record

Date Started	Medication Name	Dosage and Directions	Comments

Record of Health Care Professionals

Doctor/Provider Name	Address	Telephone Number

Helpful Questions for MTBI Survivors, Family Members, and Caregivers

1. What are the three most important things you would like your family to understand about your injury?

   A. _____

   B. _____

   C. _____

2. What things can your family do to help with your recovery?

   • Allow you to rest/sleep more.
   • Remind you not to push your limits.
   • Keep the TV, radio, voices, and other noise down.
   • Talk less to decrease overstimulation.
   • Repeat information, write it down, and talk more slowly to help with comprehension and memory.
   • Help you program devices (alarm, cell phone, PDA, etc.) which can be used for reminders, organize information (schedule, phone numbers, etc.), and help you set up and use an appointment book.
   • Help you set up a routine to structure your time.
   • Help remind you of important appointments.

- Help you find professionals to assist in your recovery, and help set up your appointments.
- Drive you to appointments, and attend your appointments with you.
- Help you look into public transportation options.
- Take you to shop and run errands or go for you.
- Help to plan and prepare meals.
- Help clean up your room, apartment or home.
- Assist with childcare.
- Assist with financial matters (e.g., paying bills, balancing checkbook, making a budget, etc.).
- Help you to understand the insurance benefits and to organize medical provider and insurance statements to alleviate confusion and frustration.
- Assist in filling our forms.
- Help you initiate your homework and other tasks.
- Assist you with your cognitive exercises (paper/pencil or computer).
- Proofread forms, checks, homework, anything that requires accuracy, to prevent mistakes.
- Read information on brain injuries to become educated about your symptoms.
- Other: _____

Hopefully, the suggested questions above will also stimulate your own creative solutions to unique situations that may arise.

Endnotes and References

We have chosen to document references to studies that are quoted in the text to make it easier for the reader. These references that are presented in chronological order by chapters are extensive enough to expand your knowledge of relevant information.

Chapter 1. Understanding Mild Traumatic Brain Injury

1. Goldstein, M. 1990. Traumatic Brain Injury: A Silent Epidemic. *Annals of Neurology* 27(3): 327.

2. Hagerman, E. 2008. Blast trauma. *Popular Science* 49-53.

3. Erichsen, J. E. 1882. *Nervous Shock and Other Obscure Injuries of the Nervous System and their Clinical Medical and Legal Aspects.* London: Longmans, Green and Company.

4. Packard, R. C. 1993. Mild head injury. *Headache Quarterly* 4(1): 42-52.

Chapter 2. Post Traumatic Stress Disorder (PTSD)

1. Russoniello, C., M. Fish, J. Parks, J. Rhodes, B. Stover, et. al. 2009. Training for optimal performance biofeedback program: A cooperative program between East Carolina University and the United States Marine Corps Wounded Warrior Battalion East. *Biofeedback* 37(1): 12-17.

2. Levine, P. A. and A. Frederick. 1997. *Waking the Tiger: Healing Trauma: The Innate Capacity to Transform Overwhelming Experiences.* Berkeley: North Atlantic, 100.

3. Levine, P. A. and A. Frederick. 1997. *Waking the Tiger: Healing Trauma: The Innate Capacity to Transform Overwhelming Experiences.* Berkeley: North Atlantic, 157.

Chapter 3. What are the Signs and Symptoms of MTBI?

1. Turk, D. C. and F. Winter. 2005. *The Pain Survival Guide: How to Reclaim Your Life.* Washington, D.C.: American Psychological Association.

2. Serrano-Duenas, M. 2005. High altitude headache. A prospective study of its clinical characteristics. *Cephalgia* 25(12): 1110-1116 and Queiroz, L. P., A. Rapoport. 2007. High altitude headaches. *Current Pain and Headache Reports* 11(4).

3. When changes in barometric pressure occur, individuals with MTBI complain of headaches intensifying.... For more information about this service, click on www.ec.gc.ca/Envirozine.

4. Belmont, A., N. Agar, C. Hugeron, B. Gallals, P. Azouvl. 2008. Fatigue and traumatic brain injury. *Ann Readapt Med Phys.* 49(6): 283-8.

5. Ouellet, M. C., C. M. Morin, A. Lavoie. 2006. Fatigue Following Traumatic Brain Injury: Frequency, Characteristics and Associated Factors. *Rehabilitation Psychology* 51(2): 140-149.

6. Johansson, B., P. Berglund, L. Ronnback. 2009. Mental fatigue and impaired information processing after mild and moderate traumatic brain injury. *Brain Injury* 23(13-14): 1027-40.

7. Cantor, J. B., T. Ashman, W. Gordon, A. Ginsberg, C. Engmann, M. Egan, L. Spielman, M. Dljkers, S. Flanagan. 2008. Fatigue after traumatic brain injury and its impact on participation and quality of life. *J Head Trauma Rehabil.* 23(1): 41-51.

8. Ziino, C. and J. Ponsford. 2006. Selective attention deficits and subjective fatigue following traumatic brain injury. *Neuropsychology* 20(3): 383-90.

9. Kohl, A. D., G. R. Wylie, H. M. Genova, F. G. Hillary, J. DeLuca. 2009. The neural correlates of cognitive fatigue in trumatic brain injury using functional MRI. *Brain Injury* 23(5): 420-432.

10. Tanriverdi, F., K. Unluhizarci, F. Kelestimur. 2009. Pituitary function in subjects with mild traumatic brain injury: a review of literature and proposal of a screening strategy. Dec. 27 Epub ahead of print.

11. Ronnback, L. and E. Hannsson. 2004. On the potential role of glutamate transport in mental fatigue, *Journal of Neuroinflammation.* 1(22): 1-9.

Chapter 4. Sports Related Concussions

1. U. S. Centers for Disease Control (CDC). 2007. Nonfatal traumatic brain injuries from sports and recreation activities. *MMWR Weekly* 56(29): 733-737.

2. Gregory, S. 2010. The problem with football. Our favorite sport is too dangerous. How to make the game safer. *TIME Magazine* 175(5): 36-43.

3. McKee, A. 2009. Hearing before the House judiciary Committee: Legal issues relating to football head injuries. *Written Testimony* October 28, 2009 1-13.

4. Tommasone, B. and T. Valovich-McLeod. 2006. Contact sport concussion incidence. *J of Athletic Training* 41(4): 470-472.

5. Kelly J. P. and J. H. Rosenberg. 1997. The diagnosis and management of concussion in sports. *Neurology* 48: 575-580.

6. Kelly, J. P. and J. H. Rosenberg. 1997. Practice Parameter: The management of concussion in sports. *Neurology* 48: 581-585.

7. Kelly, J. P. and J. H. Rosenberg. 1997. Practice Parameter: The management of concussion in sports. *Neurology.* 48: 581-585.

8. For more information, click on www.headinjury.com/sports.htm

9. Schwarz A. Girls are often neglected victims of concussions *New York Times,* October 2, 2007.

10. Yeoman, B. December 2004. Lights Out: Can contact sports lower your intelligence? *Discover* 68-73.

11. High-tech football helmets reveal new information about head injuries. College of Arts and Sciences, University of North Carolina, Chapel Hill. December 2007. http://college.unc.edu/features/december2007-12-07.0451328104

12. Sports-related recurrent brain injuries. CNN, *Sports Illustrated* (CNNSI.com), July, 1999.

13. Gregory, S. 2010. The problem with football. *TIME Magazine* 175(5): 36-42.

Chapter 5. The Important Role of Brain Filters

1. *Mayo Clinic Health Letter* December, 1994. 12(12).

Chapter 10. Feed Your Body, Feed Your Brain

1. Jay, G. 2000. *Minor Traumatic Brain Injury Handbook: Diagnosis and Treatment.* New York: CRC Press.

Chapter 11. How To Improve Memory and Thinking Skills

1. Ratey, J. and E. Hagerman. 2008. *Spark: The Revolutionary New Science of Exercise and the Brain.* New York: Little, Brown and Company.

Chapter 12. What is Biofeedback and Neurofeedback?

1. Ayres, M. 1987. Electroencephalographic Neurofeedback and Closed Head Injury, Head Injury Frontier, National Head Injury Foundation Annual Conference 380-392. Bounias, M., R. G. Laibow, A. Bonaly, et. al. 2001. EEG Neurofeedback Treatment of Patients with Brain Injury, Part 1: Typographical Clarification of Clinical Syndromes. *Journal of Neurotherapy* 5(4): 23-44. Thornton, K. 2000. Improvements/Rehabilitation of Memory Functioning with Neurotherapy/QEEG Biofeedback. *Journal of Head Trauma Rehabiliation* 15(6): 1285-1296.

2. Thornton, K and D. Carmody. 2008. Efficacy of traumatic brain injury rehabilitation: Interventions of QEEG-guided biofeedback, computers, strategies and medications. *Applied Psychophysiology and Biofeedback* 33(2): 101-124.

3. Duff, J. 2004. The usefulness of QEEG and neurotherapy in the assessment and treatment of post-concussion syndrome. *Clinical EEG Neuroscience* 35(4): 198-209.

4. Russoniello, C., M. Fish, J. Parks, et. al. 2009. Training for optimal performance biofeedback program: A cooperative program between East Carolina University and the United States Marine Corps Wounded Warrior Battalion East. *Biofeedback* 37(1): 12-17.

5. Peniston, E. G. and P. J. Kulkosky. 1991. Alpha-theta brainwave neurofeedback therapy for vietnam veterans with combat-related post-traumatic stress dis-order. *Medical Psychotherapy, An International Journal* 4: 47-60.

Chapter 16. What's the Good News?

1. Restak, R. 2001. *Mozart's Brain and the Fighter Pilot.* New York: Harmony Press.

2. Braverman, E. 2004. *The Edge Effect: Reverse or Prevent Alzheimer's, Aging, Memory Loss, Weight Gain, Sexual Dysfunction, and More.* New York: Sterling Publishing Company, Inc.

3. N. Doidge. 2007. *The Brain That Changes Itself: Stories of Personal Triumph from the Frontiers of Brain Science.* New York: Viking.

Resources

Recommended Head Injury Web Sites

www.ablelinktech.com

Offers resources in assistive technology for individuals with intellectual and cognitive disabilities, such as software packages that interface with handheld PCs.

www.ASHA.org

The American Speech-Language Hearing Association maintains this website to help you locate cognitive therapists and speech/language pathologists in your area.

www.bcia.org.

Biofeedback Certification International Alliance. Helps you locate certified biofeedback practitioners.

www.biausa.org
Brain Injury Association of America can direct you to local offices in your area. Search their website for other resources including location of neuropractitioners in your area.

www.biacolorado.org
Brain Injury Association of Colorado.

www.braininjury.com
A medical, legal, and informational resource for persons dealing with traumatic brain injury.

www.braininjurychat.org
Peer Support for people living with brain injury.

www.brainline.org
Resources for preventing, treating and living with TBI.

www.cdc.gov/concussion/HeadsUp/youth.html
An online source for credible health information and a tool kit about preventing concussions in youth sports.

www.eeginfo.com
A website with information about neurofeedback.

www.emdr.com
Learn about eye movement desensitization and reprocessing (EMDR). It has been proven to produce profound treatment effects in eliminating or greatly diminishing the emotional distress related to a traumatic memory. Clients who experience the EMDR processing also gain important cognitive insights.

www.foodsafety.gov
Ideas for practicing safe handling of food.

www.freedomdogs.org
Freedom Dogs offers custom-trained specialty service dogs to wounded members of the military returning from armed conflict.

www.FreeHearingTest.com offers an online, free hearing test. The site is a convenient compilation of hearing healthcare resources and information.

www.headinjury.com
This is a nonprofit organization with an abundance of information to build skills and to participate in discussion groups. You can also link to resources, rehab, and research sites for all types of head injuries.

www.hearplugz.com Learn about a multi-functional dual filtered hearing protector that allows you to hear critical sounds needed for communication and environmental awareness. It is one of the product developed by the Environmental Acoustical Research, Inc., **www.earinc.com**.

www.Independentliving.com Information about assistive devices that can help compensate for cognitive deficits, such as impaired memory and disorientation to time range from simple appointment books and basic digital watches with alarm function to more advanced devices, such as vibrating watches which display messages.

www.sharpbrains.com
SharpBrains provides independent, research-based, information and guidance to navigate the growing cognitive and brain fitness market.

www.traumahealing.com
Learn about Somatic Experiencing® which is a body-awareness approach to trauma being taught throughout the world. It is the result of over forty years of observation, research, and hands-on development by Dr. Peter Levine.

www.waiting.com. We are not medical professionals; however we encourage your inquiries regarding legal issues and information on further resources. Phone and email inquiries will be received by the staff of the Brain Injury Law Office, including Attorney Gordon S. Johnson, Jr.

The following websites are used to improve cognitive functioning:

> **www.puzzlersparadise.com**
> **www.CogniFit.com**
> **www.braingle.com**
> **www.Lumosity.com**

Recommended Books

Being a Brain-Wise Therapist: A Practical Guide to Interpersonal Neurobiology (Norton Series on Interpersonal Neurobiology), by Bonnie Badenoch. New York: W. W. Norton & Co, 2008.

Brain Injury Survival Kit: 365 Tips, Tools & Tricks to Deal with Cognitive Function Loss, by Cheryl Sullivan. New York: Demo Medical Publishing, 2008.

Brain Injury Survivor's Guide: Welcome to Our World, Larry Jameson and Beth Jameson. Parker: *Outskirts Press, 2007.*

Change Your Brain, Change Your Life, by Daniel G. Amen, New York: Three Rivers Press, 1998.

Healing Trauma: A Pioneering Program for Restoring the Wisdom of Your Body, by Peter A. Levine, PhD. Louisville: Sounds True, 2008.

If Only I'd Had this Caregiving Book, by Maya Hennessey. Bloomington: AuthorHouse, 2006.

I'll Carry the Fork: Recovering a Life After Brain Injury, by Kara L. Swanson. Scotts Valley: Rising Star Press, 1999.

Keep your Brain Alive: 83 Neurobic Exercises to Help Prevent Memory Loss and Increase Mental Fitness, by Lawrence C. Katz, PhD and Manning Rubin. New York: Workman Publishing, 1999.

Magnificent Mind At Any Age: Treat Anxiety, Depression, Memory Problems, ADD, and Insomnia, by Daniel G. Amen, MD. New York: Harmony Books, 2008.

Mild Traumatic Brain Injury: A Clinician's Guide, Edited by Michael J. Raymond, Thomas L. Bennett, Laurence C. Hartlage and C. Munro Cullum. Austin: Pro-ed Publishers, 1999.

My Stroke of Insight: A Brain Scientist's Personal Journey, by Jill Bolte Taylor, PhD. New York: Viking Penguin, 2008.

Spark: The Revolutionary New Science of Exercise and the Brain, by John J. Ratey, MD. New York: Little, Brown and Company, 2008.

The Body Bears the Burden: Trauma, Dissociation, and Disease, by Robert C. Scaer, MD, PhD. Binghamton: Da Capo Press, 2008.

The Brain That Changes Itself, by Norman Doidge, MD. New York: Viking Penguin, 2007.

The Chronic Pain Care Workbook: A Self-Treatment Approach to Pain Relief Using the Behavioral Assessment of Pain Questionnaire, by Michael J. Lewandowski, PhD. Oakland, CA: New Haringer Publications, Inc., 2006.

The Edge Effect: Reverse or Prevent Alzheimer's, Aging, Memory Loss, Weight Gain, Sexual Dysfunction, and More, by Eric R. Braverman, MD. New York: Sterling Publishing Co., Inc., 2004.

The Evaluation and Treatment of Mild Traumatic Brain Injury, edited by Nils R. Varney and Richard J. Roberts. Lawrence Erlbaum. Mahwah: Associated Publishers, 1999.

The Pain Survival Guide: How to Reclaim Your Life, by Dennis C. Turk and Fritz Winter, PhD. Washington, D.C.: American Psychological Association, 2005.

The Scientific American Brave New Brain: How Neuroscience, Brain-Machine Interfaces, Neuroimaging, Psychopharmacology, Epignetics, the Internet and Our Minds Are Stimulating and Enhancing the Future of Mental Power, by Judith Horstman and Scientific American. New York: Jossey-Bass, 2010.

The Sharp Brains Guide to Brain Fitness: 18 Interviews with Scientists, Practical Advice, and Product Reviews, to Keep Your Brain Sharp by Alvaro Fernandez and Dr. Elkhonon Goldberg. San Francisco: SharpBrains, 2009.

Waking the Tiger: Healing Trauma: the Innate Capacity to Transform Overwhelming Experiences, by Peter A. Levine and Ann Frederick. Berkeley: North Atlantic Books, 1997.

Your Miracle Brain: Dramatic New Scientific Evidence Reveals How You Can Use Food and Supplements to: Maximize your Brainpower, Boost Your Memory, Lift Your Mood, Improve Your IQ and Creativity, and Prevent and Reverse Mental Aging, by Jean Carper. New York: Harper Collins, 2001.

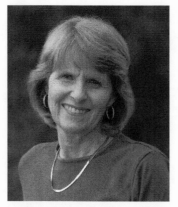Mary Ann Keatley, PhD, CCC, is a speech-language pathologist and neurotherapist who has specialized in the treatment of traumatic brain injuries and other neurological conditions for more than 30 years. Her broad experience includes neurorehabilitation, research, and publications in the fields of speech-language pathology, rehabilitation, and outcomes. She is a professional speaker and gives presentations and training in the field of brain injuries and recovery, and has a private practice in Boulder, Colorado. She is the co-founder of the Brain Injury Hope Foundation.

Laura L. Whittemore has been in the field of psychology and education and has been an entrepreneur for more than 30 years. She sustained a TBI in 2001, caused by a horseback riding accident. Fortunately, she was wearing a helmet. Since her life-changing, wake 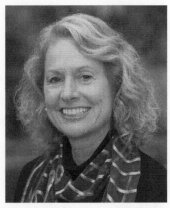 up call, she has focused her gifts gained through her recovery process into writing, speaking, life coaching, and creating memory fitness programs. Laura has two children and six grandchildren and lives, hikes, and skis in sunny Colorado.

HOW TO ORDER

Online Orders: www.BrainInjuryHopeFoundation.org
Telephone Orders: 303-484-2126
Email Contact: info@BrainInjuryHopeFoundation.org

Understanding Mild Traumatic Brain Injury(MTBI):
An Insightful Guide to Symptoms, Treatments and
Redefining Recovery...$14.95

Also, please consider buying the following book for a Wounded
Warrior that you may know.

Recovering from Mild Traumatic Brain Injury (MTBI:
A Handbook of Hope for Our Military Warriors and
Their Families..$12.95

Sales Tax: Please add 3% for books shipped to Colorado addresses.

Shipping: Please add $3.50 for the first book and $1.50 for
each additional book. Please call or email for shipping rates
for quantities of books over five.

Ask for Quantity Discounts starting at 25 books.

Proceeds from book sales go to the non-profit:

**Brain Injury Hope Foundation
P.O. Box 1319
Boulder, CO 80306**

Made in the USA
San Bernardino, CA
18 October 2013